Key advances in
the effective management

of

Unstable Angina

Edited by
J Ferguson and H Purcell

Series Organiz
A Miles

GW00702928

*Proceedings of a symposium sponsored by Pharmacia & Upjohn Ltd and held at the
Royal Society of Medicine, London, 19th October 1998*

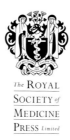

The ROYAL
SOCIETY *of*
MEDICINE
PRESS *Limited*

1 Wimpole Street, London W1M 8AE, UK
207 E. Westminster Road, Lake Forest, IL 60045, USA
http://www.roysocmed.ac.uk

These proceedings are published by the Royal Society of Medicine Press Ltd with
financial support from the sponsor. The contributors are responsible for the scientific
content and for the views expressed, which are not necessarily those of the editor of
the series or of the volume, of the Royal Society of Medicine or of the Royal Society of
Medicine Press Ltd. Distribution has been in accordance with the wishes of the
sponsor but a copy is available to any fellow of the society at a privileged price.

British Library Cataloguing in Publication Data

A catalogue record for this book is available from the British Library

ISBN 1–85315–391–5

Typeset by Saxon Graphics Ltd, Derby

Printed in Great Britain by Latimer Trend & Company Ltd, Plymouth

Editors

Dr John Ferguson
Prescription Pricing Authority, Bridge House,
152 Pilgrim Street, Newcastle upon Tyne NE1 6SN

Dr Henry Purcell
Royal Brompton and Harefield NHS Trust,
Sydney Street, London SW3 6NP

Contributors

Dr Nicholas Curzen
Manchester Heart Centre,
Manchester Royal Infirmary, Manchester M13 9WL

Dr Miles Dalby
Royal Brompton and Harefield NHS Trust,
Sydney Street, London SW3 6NP

Mr John Dunning
Papworth Hospital NHS Trust, Papworth, Everard,
Cambridge CB3 8RE

Dr Kim Fox
Royal Brompton and Harefield NHS Trust,
Sydney Street, London SW3 6NP

Dr Robert Henderson
Nottingham City Hospital,
Hucknall Road, Nottingham NG5 1PB

Dr Diana Holdright
The Middlesex Hospital, Mortimer Street, London W1N 8AA

Dr Simon Kennon
Southend General Hospital,
Prittlewell Chase, Westcliffe-on-Sea, Essex SS0 0RY

Dr Govindaraj Mohan
James Paget Hospital NHS Trust, Lowestoft Road, Gorleston
Great Yarmouth, Norfolk NR31 6LA

Dr Martin Rothman
The London Chest Hospital,
Bonner Road, London E2 9JX

Dr Mary Sheppard
Royal Brompton and Harefield NHS Trust,
Sydney Street, London SW3 6NP

Dr Adam Timmis
The London Chest Hospital,
Bonner Road, London E2 9JX

Contents

Foreword

The Key Advances symposia held at the Royal Society of Medicine aim to provide a solidly clinical contribution to evidence-based medicine in the UK. Attention is focused on open debate and the contextual interpretation of new medical evidence in a variety of common disease states.

The symposia are intended to facilitate true analysis of the available evidence: practice guidelines, scientific evidence, cost-effectiveness and clinical audit data.

This book presents clinical strategies for the efficient and effective management of unstable angina. The Guest Editors and contributors, all distinguished clinicians in their field, are to be commended for their efforts in producing an accessible, highly readable text of immediate relevance to continuing medical education and personal clinical practice.

Professor Andrew Miles
Series Organizer
St Bartholomew's Hospital, London

Preface

Unstable angina is a heterogeneous condition, sometimes described as a 'halfway house' between stable angina and acute myocardial infarction (MI). It is characterized by severe myocardial ischaemia and, despite best current treatments, is still associated with high morbidity and mortality. Hospital admission rates for unstable angina have increased steadily in many countries over the past decade. Unlike stable angina, which is primarily associated with increased oxygen demand, the most important mechanism of ischaemia in unstable coronary syndromes is a primary reduction in myocardial oxygen supply due to atherosclerotic plaque disruption with associated thrombosis and vasoconstriction. The process of coronary plaque rupture is well described, and is a function of plaque vulnerability and 'triggers' of rupture (eg mechanical and psychological stress). Vulnerability is related to the type of plaque rather than the severity of the vessel narrowing.

The degree of obstruction caused by this superimposed, local thrombosis determines the severity of the syndrome. A non-occlusive thrombus may manifest as unstable angina, with complete occlusion often evolving into a Q wave MI, with platelets playing a central role. The unstable coronary lesion (particularly complex lesions) is often not stabilized with medical treatment and will continue to progress over ensuing months. Many opportunities exist to modify the underlying factors and triggers leading to plaque rupture, to promote passiveness of the active plaque thereby preventing reactivation, and for the use of anti-inflammatory, anti-thrombotic and lipid-lowering therapy.

This book reviews many of these new treatments in this fast-moving field, including low molecular weight heparin, clopidogrel, glycoprotein IIb/IIIa inhibitors, as well as intervention. Other important issues in the effective management of unstable angina include the economic implications of potential therapies, hospital diagnosis, and secondary preventative measures. Although these topics were presented at the symposium, unfortunately, they are not included in these proceedings.

Dr John Ferguson
Prescription Pricing Authority
Newcastle upon Tyne

Dr Henry Purcell
Royal Brompton and Harefield NHS Trust
London

Unstable angina and its causes

Henry Purcell, Miles Dalby, Mary Sheppard and Kim Fox, Royal Brompton and Harefield NHS Trust, London

Unstable angina has been described as something of a 'wastebasket' diagnosis encompassing acute coronary insufficiency, crescendo angina, preinfarction angina (retrospectively) and other, now outmoded, labels. Unstable angina consists of a number of different conditions which are characterized by severe myocardial ischaemia. An earlier classification defining unstable angina[1] has been refined as one of the following: new onset chest pain of less than one month's duration occurring with minimal exertion; acceleration of previously stable angina (more frequent and/or with less exertion) with more severe and prolonged (> 15 min) episodes that are less responsive to antianginal drugs; rest or nocturnal angina; and angina occurring or recurring less than one month after myocardial infarction or following coronary revascularization by surgery or angioplasty.[2] Diagnosis of unstable angina depends on careful physical examination and clinical history. Use of the 12-lead electrocardiogram (ECG) and measurement of cardiac enzymes (increasingly to include troponin T levels) will exclude the likelihood of Q wave myocardial infarction (MI) and will help in patient risk stratification.

Incidence and prevalence of unstable angina

Getting a clear view of the incidence and prevalence of unstable angina is not easy due to the lack of standardization in its definition and diagnosis. A specific code for unstable angina only became available in recent years within the 10th revision of the International Classification of Diseases (ICD 10).

The National Center for Health Statistics in the US recorded 750,000 admissions for unstable angina in 1993, with a further 750,000 admissions for acute myocardial infarction (AMI).[3] As one-third of these were non-Q wave MIs (NQWMI) using a broader definition, approximately one million patients were admitted to hospital with acute coronary syndromes.

US hospital discharge rates for unstable angina have shown a consistent and dramatic increase in recent years, accounting for 25% of all coronary artery disease (CAD) discharges in 1989 compared to 4% in 1980.[4] During this period, AMI rates have plateaued. This trend is unlikely to abate as almost 60% of the people admitted for unstable angina in 1993 were over 65 years of age, and this is the most rapidly growing segment of the American population.[5] Similar trends have occurred in Canada where the incidence of unstable angina and NQWMI tripled between 1985–1994, and the incidence of Q wave MI has remained relatively unchanged.[6] In Europe, the annual number of hospital admissions for acute coronary syndromes is approximately two million, more than one-half of which are for unstable angina or NQWMI.[7] As in other parts of Europe, unstable angina is one of the most common causes of admission to UK coronary care units. The magnitude of the problem may be far greater in the UK than officially recorded statistics suggest.[8] Various studies throughout the literature have recorded a higher volume of admissions for unstable angina than for AMI.

A number of factors may play a role in the apparent rise in unstable angina rates, including changes in disease coding and greater awareness of the condition generally. Lifestyle changes, such as smoking cessation and the adoption of low-fat diets and increased exercise in individuals at risk, may influence disease rates. Similarly, the increasing use of secondary prevention with HMG CoA reductase inhibitors (statins) — which may have activity independent of their lipid-lowering effects — β-blockers, angiotensin-converting enzyme (ACE) inhibitors and aspirin may also have an effect. A number of studies suggest that aspirin has the potential to produce less severe acute coronary syndromes and attenuate the underlying disease process, such that unstable angina patients taking aspirin before hospital admission

1

are less likely to present with NQWMI or Q wave MI.[9] These observations with aspirin suggest that platelets (thrombi) are a major culprit in unstable angina. Platelet activation and aggregation is a rapid process which can be demonstrated in vitro.

Causes of unstable angina

Coronary thrombosis occurs through two distinct processes.[10] First, the endothelium covering the atherosclerotic plaque becomes denuded or eroded and a thrombus is superimposed on the plaque surface. Second, plaque disruption occurs with the tearing open of the fibrous cap to expose the highly thrombogenic lipid core; approximately 75% of thrombi responsible for acute coronary syndromes are precipitated in this way. Some plaque disruption may cause minor fissures. The extent to which the superimposed thrombus obstructs coronary blood flow and its effect on the myocardium determines the development of unstable angina or AMI,[11] and symptoms occur when major intraluminal thrombi develop (Figure 1). The sequence of events from endothelial dysfunction and the appearance of the fatty streak (the earliest lesion of atherosclerosis) through to the development of the mature plaque (which may take 10–15 years), plaque rupture and coronary thrombosis, has been well characterized through the work of Michael Davies, Erling Falk and others.[12,13]

Plaque rupture depends more on the type of plaque than its size. The major determinants of plaque vulnerability are:

- the size and consistency of the atheromatous core
- the thickness of the fibrous plaque
- ongoing inflammation and repair within the cap.

Plaque shape is a further consideration. Acute coronary syndromes are more frequently associated with eccentric (as distinct from concentric) stenoses which form an arc-shaped

Figure 1: Perfused, fixed human coronary artery in an unstable angina patient showing ruptured plaque with superimposed non-occlusive intraluminal thrombus

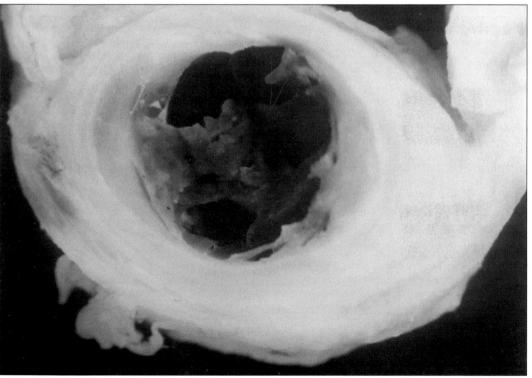

lumen. Local factors such as shear forces, coronary tone and pressure, as well as the bending and twisting of the artery with cardiac contractility, also influence susceptibility to fissuring.[14] Coronary spasm may also contribute to the development of myocardial ischaemia. A number of physical 'triggers', such as exertion in normally sedentary individuals, have been identified as causing acute coronary events. Patients hospitalized for acute coronary syndromes have, on average, signficantly higher levels of psychological distress than controls, which supports the concept that emotional life events may also act as triggers of acute ischaemia.[15]

Atherosclerotic plaques prone to rupture have a large, lipid-rich pool, with less collagen but with a heavy inflammatory component; plaques with a lipid core comprising >40% of the overall plaque volume are particularly susceptible to rupture. Angiotensin II has been shown to co-localize with macrophages in the intima-media layers of atherosclerotic plaques.[16] All these factors may contribute to vascular dysfunction through the stimulation of smooth muscle cell proliferation, and increasing the accumulation of cholesterol and the formation of foam cells.

The fibrous plaque, comprising collagen-rich fibrous tissue containing smooth muscle cells, stands between the lipid core and the blood. Plaque rupture frequently occurs at the vulnerable shoulder region where the cap is thin and acellular (Figure 2). The macrophages and smooth muscle cells secrete matrix metalloproteinases (MMPs) which regulate degradation of the extracellular matrix, leading to collagen fragmentation and cap weakening.[17] In addition, macrophages express tissue factor which is a major thrombogenic stimulus. Mast cells within the plaque also contribute to matrix degradation.[18] Inflammation is associated with increased production of acute phase proteins, and an increased circulating concentration of C-reactive protein is a predictor of coronary events in patients with stable and unstable angina.[19] Interaction between leucocytes and endothelial cells is also important in inflammation. Such interaction is regulated by cell adhesion molecules. Significantly greater expression of the adhesion molecule P-selectin was found from atherectomy samples in patients with unstable angina.[20] It is also feasible that infectious processes contribute to inflammation and plaque instability in acute coronary syndromes.[21]

Figure 2: Histological section of human coronary artery showing disruption at cap shoulder. The area above the fissure site is thrombus

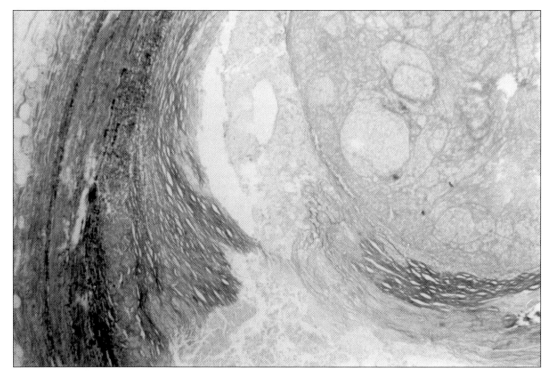

The potential significance of reducing the inflammatory milieu is underlined by two recent studies. Lipid lowering by diet reduces MMP activity and increases interstitial collagen, thereby providing lesion stabilization in rabbits.[22] Reduction of inflammation with pravastatin is associated with a reduced risk of coronary events in post-MI patients with average cholesterol levels.[23] Clearly, other pharmacological interventions may also lead to plaque stabilization.

Many advanced plaques are not angiographically visible and fissuring frequently occurs in areas with a <50% pre-existing stenosis: this also supports the notion that plaque disruption is related more to the type of plaque than the severity of the luminal narrowing.[24] Angiographically complex lesions are associated with an adverse result which is not often medically stabilized and will continue to progress over the ensuing months.[25] Angioscopic studies confirm that a thrombus is non-occlusive in 80% of patients with unstable angina and that it is composed primarily of platelets, in contrast to AMI in which occlusive red, fibrin-rich thrombi predominate.[26] Angioscopy has also shown that an active, unstable plaque is clearly visible more than one month after AMI.[27] Such findings suggest the need for more potent and prolonged antiplatelet therapy after an acute ischaemic event.

Continuous ST segment (Holter) monitoring in treated unstable angina shows that episodes of transient myocardial ischaemia, occurring predominantly at night, are invariably not preceded by an increase in heart rate.[28] This suggests that the ischaemia relates primarily to a reduction in myocardial oxygen supply due to a non-occlusive mural thrombus (as described above) at the time of reduced endogenous fibrinolytic activity. A greater increase in the morning incidence of unstable angina with exertional pain compared with rest pain is observed between 6 am and 12 noon.[29] Such circadian patterns in myocardial ischaemia may also have important bearings on patient management.

Conclusion

The incidence of unstable angina appears to be increasing. Prognosis is not benign and an increased understanding of this, primarily thrombus-driven, condition may have important implications for improving symptoms and outcome.

References

1. Braunwald E. Unstable angina. A classification. *Circulation* 1989; **80**: 410–4.
2. von Dohlen TW, Rogers WB, Frank MJ. Pathophysiology and management of unstable angina. *Clin Cardiol* 1989; **12**: 363–9.
3. Collins JG. *Prevalence of selected chronic conditions. United States, 1986–88*. Washington: US Government Printing Office. National Center for Health Statistics, Vital and Health Statistics, 1993; DHHS publication no. (PHS)93–1510.
4. Whitney EJ, Shear CL, Mantell G *et al.* The case for unstable angina pectoris as a primary end point in primary prevention studies. *Am J Cardiol* 1992; **70**: 738–43.
5. Eisenstein EL. Patient risk or physician practice: What factors drive resource use in unstable angina? *Am Heart J* 1998; **13**: 365–7.
6. Montague T, Montague P, Barnes M *et al.* Acute myocardial infarction in Canada: New epidemiologic insights on incidence, therapy and risk. *J Thromb Thrombol* 1996; **3**: 101–5.
7. Neuhhaus KL. *Coronary thrombosis-defining the goals, improving the outcome*. Presentation during XVIIIth Congress, European Society of Cardiology, 25 August 1996.
8. Purcell H. The epidemiology of unstable angina. *Br J Cardiol* 1998; **5**(suppl 2): S3–4.
9. Garcia-Dorado D, Théroux P, Tornos P *et al.* Previous aspirin use may attenuate the severity of the manifestation of acute ischaemic syndromes. *Circulation* 1995; **92**: 1743–8.
10. Davies MJ. The role of plaque pathology in coronary thrombosis. *Clin Cardiol* 1997; **20**(suppl 1): 1–2Ô1–7.
11. Davies MJ, Woolf N. Atherosclerosis: what is it and why does it occur? *Br Heart J* 1993; **69**(suppl): S3–11.
12. Davies MJ, Thomas AC. Plaque fissuring – the cause of acute myocardial infarction, sudden ischaemic death, and crescendo angina. *Br Heart J* 1985; **53**: 363–73.
13. Falk E. Unstable angina with fatal outcome; dynamic cornary thrombosis leading to infarction and/or sudden death. *Circulation* 1985; **71**: 699–708.

14. Fuster V, Badimon L, Badimon JJ, Chesebro JH. The pathogenesis of coronary artery disease and the acute coronary syndromes. *N Engl J Med* 1992; **326**: 242–50.

15. Pignalberi C, Patti G, Chimenti C *et al*. Role of different determinants of psychological distress in acute coronary syndromes. *J Am Coll Cardiol* 1998; **32**: 613–9.

16. Potter DD, Sobey CG, Tompkins PK *et al*. Evidence that macrophages in atherosclerotic lesions contain angiotensin II. *Circulation* 1998; **98**: 800–7.

17. Kai H, Ikeda H, Yasukawa H *et al*. Peripheral blood levels of matrix metalloproteinases-2 and -9 are elevated in patients with acute coronary syndromes. *J Am Coll Cardiol* 1998; **32**: 368–72.

18. Kaartinen M, Van der Wal, Van der Loos CM *et al*. Mast cell infiltration in acute coronary syndromes: Implications for plaque rupture. *J Am Coll Cardiol* 1998; **32**: 606–12.

19. Haverkate F, Thompson SG, Pyke SDM *et al* for the European Concerted Action on Thrombosis and Disabilities Angina Pectoris Study Group. *Lancet* 1997; **349**: 462–6.

20. Tenaglia AN, Buda AJ, Wilkins RG *et al*. Levels of expression of P-selectin, E-selectin and intercellular adhesion molecule-1 in coronary atherectomy specimens from patients with stable and unstable angina. *Am J Cardiol* 1997; **79**: 742–7.

21. Gurfinkel E, Bozovich G, Daroca A *et al*. Randomised trial of roxithromycin in non-Q wave coronary syndromes: ROXIS pilot study. *Lancet* 1997; **350**: 404–7.

22. Aikawa M, Rabkin E, Okada Y *et al*. Lipid lowering by diet reduces matrix metalloproteinase activity and increases collagen content of rabbit atheroma. *Circulation* 1998; **97**: 2433–44.

23. Ridker PM, Rifai N, Pfeffer MA *et al*. Inflammation, pravastatin, and the risk of coronary events after myocardial infarction in patients with average cholesterol levels. *Circulation* 1998; **98**: 839–44.

24. Ribeiro PA, Shah PM. Unstable angina: New insights into pathophysiologic characteristics, prognosis, and management strategies. *Curr Probl Cardiol* 1996; **21**: 675–731.

25. Chen L, Chester MR, Redwood S *et al*. Angiographic stenosis progression and coronary events in patients with 'stabilised' unstable angina. *Circulation* 1995; **91**: 2319–24.

26. Mizuno K, Satomura K, Miyamoto A *et al*. Angioscopic evaluation of coronary-artery thrombi in acute coronary syndromes. *N Engl J Med* 1992; **326**: 287–91.

27. Van Belle E, Lablanche J-M, Bauters C *et al*. Coronary angioscopic findings in the infarct-related vessel within 1 month of acute myocardial infarction. *Circulation* 1998; **97**: 26–33.

28. Patel DJ, Knight CJ, Holdright DR *et al*. Pathophysiology of transient myocardial ischemia in acute coronary syndromes. *Circulation* 1997; **95**: 1185–92.

29. Cannon CP, McCabe CH, Stone PH *et al*. Circadian variation in the onset of unstable angina and non-Q wave acute myocardial infarction (the TIMI III Registry and TIMI IIIB). *Am J Cardiol* 1997; **79**: 253–8.

Clinical predictors of presentation: unstable angina or myocardial infarction

Adam Timmis, London Chest Hospital, London
Simon Kennon, Southend General Hospital, Essex

Unstable angina and myocardial infarction (MI) are two acute coronary syndromes that share a common pathogenesis in the rupture of atherosclerotic plaques, followed by the formation of intraluminal thrombi as a result of the exposure of plaque contents to blood. The clinical presentation of plaque rupture is determined by several factors and these will be outlined in this paper.

Thrombosis

Thrombosis occurs as a result of the interaction between three systems: platelets (activation and aggregation), the coagulation cascade and the vascular endothelium.

Platelet activation and aggregation

Intraluminal thrombi consist of platelets bound together with insoluble fibrin strands, thereby forming a plug. Under physiological conditions, platelets do not adhere to each other, intact endothelial cells, or other blood constituents — they are maintained in this resting state by prostacyclin and nitric oxide, which are secreted by the vascular endothelium. Platelets must be activated for aggregation to occur.

Activation occurs in the presence of several platelet agonists, the most important of which include collagen (present following plaque rupture), thromboxane (released by activated platelets) and thrombin (a product of the coagulation cascade).[1] Activation involves the expression of the fibrinogen receptor — glycoprotein IIb/IIIa — on the platelet surface. This receptor also plays a role in platelet interaction with neutrophils, endothelial cells and clotting factors, and in platelet degranulation, which causes the release of the potent, chemo-attractants, inflammatory mediators and coagulation factors involved in the final common pathway of the coagulation cascade.

Fibrin formation

Following plaque rupture, tissue factor (present in the atheromatous core of the plaque) interacts with factor VII — this initiates the formation of thrombin via the coagulation cascade. Thrombin acts on fibrinogen and converts it to fibrin which, in turn, is degraded by plasmin. The conversion of plasmin from its inactive precursor, plasminogen, is regulated by the balance between tissue plasminogen activator and plasminogen activator inhibitor 1 levels, but mainly by the latter (an enzyme produced and secreted by the vascular endothelium).[2]

Vascular endothelium

The vascular endothelium produces a number of other substances important in vascular homeostasis and cardiovascular pathophysiology, including endothelins, thromboxane A_2 and von Willebrand factor. The vascular endothelium, therefore, controls vascular tone, fibrin deposition and lysis, as well as leucocyte and platelet activation. Its dysfunction is associated with atherogenesis, vasospasm and a prothrombotic state.[3,4]

Consequences of thrombosis

Platelet activation is, therefore, vital not only for platelet aggregation but also for fibrin deposition and plug formation. Fibrin strengthens the platelet plug by capturing erythrocytes and binding platelets together to form intraluminal thrombi which restrict blood flow.[5] If the thrombus is sufficiently large to cause artery occlusion and thus interruption of the blood supply to an area of myocardium, necrosis of that area occurs — this characterizes the condition of acute MI. In unstable angina, however, the thrombus is transient or subocclusive, and low-grade perfusion of the myocardium at risk is maintained.[6,7]

Determinants of clinical presentation

Although plaque rupture initiates thrombosis, it is frequently not marked by a clinical event but is 'silent'.[8] Despite obvious prognostic implications, little research has been carried out to determine what dictates the clinical presentation of plaque rupture. Clearly, the magnitude of the thrombotic response to plaque rupture is important and is determined by the extent of the thrombogenic stimulus and prevailing systemic propensity to thrombosis. The size of the thrombogenic stimulus has been shown to be related to a number of factors, such as degree of plaque disruption, nature of the thrombogenic substrate and local blood flow conditions.[9]

Nature of the plaque

Atherosclerotic plaques do not rupture spontaneously but in response to triggering forces — in addition, certain plaques are more vulnerable to rupture than others. Such vulnerable plaques have large, lipid-rich cores containing numerous inflammatory cells and are covered by a thin, fibrous cap.[10] The lipid-rich core is the most thrombogenic component of the plaque and has a low mechanical strength threshold, hence its high vulnerability.[11] Lipid-lowering therapies reduce the lipid content of the plaque, producing stronger, more stable and, presumably, less thrombogenic plaques.[12]

Mechanical forces

Plaque rupture can be triggered by physical and emotional stress as a result of increased blood and pulse pressures, heart rate and coronary tone. Plaque rupture that leads to a high degree of stenosis and surface irregularity results in high blood velocity and shear forces that lead to shear-induced platelet activation. This process is unique as it involves the binding of only one protein — von Willebrand factor — to platelet glycoprotein Ib and is independent of the usual range of activating agents, including thromboxane A_2.[13]

Haemostatic factors

The systemic propensity to thrombosis depends on the prevailing balance between prothrombotic and anti-thrombotic forces. Thrombolytic therapy helps to restore coronary flow in acute MI, while heparin and aspirin protect against thrombotic occlusion in unstable angina.[14] Such treatment, applied after the plaque event, has significantly improved the prognosis of these coronary syndromes by reducing or preventing myocardial necrosis. If therapeutic modification of thrombotic responses to plaque rupture favourably influences the natural history of acute coronary syndromes, it is possible that the mode of presentation itself might be influenced by the balance between prothrombotic and anti-thrombotic activity at the time of the plaque event. Factors that increase thrombotic responses to plaque rupture could, therefore, favour presentation with MI rather than unstable angina and, conversely, factors that reduce the thrombotic response favour presentation with unstable angina.

This hypothesis was tested by logging clinical characteristics of a consecutive series of 1,111 patients diagnosed with unstable angina ($n=478$) and MI ($n=633$), who were admitted to our coronary care unit. Table 1 summarizes the results of the multivariate analysis, which are discussed overleaf.[15]

Table 1 Multivariate predictors of discharge diagnosis. Odds ratios (ORs) represent the odds of myocardial infarction relative to unstable angina

	OR	95% CI	p value
Age (years)			
<50	1.0		
50–59	0.98	0.59–1.62	
60–69	1.18	0.73–1.92	
>70	2.21	1.33–3.66	0.001 (for trend)
Gender			
female	1.0		
male	1.56	1.13–2.16	0.008
Smoking	1.49	1.09–2.03	0.013
Hypertension	0.64	0.47–0.86	0.004
Diabetes	0.97	0.70–1.36	0.87
Drugs on admission			
aspirin	0.37	0.27–0.52	<0.001
β-blocker	0.79	0.53–1.18	0.25
Previous acute coronary syndromes	0.36	0.26–0.51	<0.001
Previous revascularization	0.36	0.21–0.62	<0.001
Admission biochemistry			
potassium	0.78	0.56–1.10	0.20
creatinine	1.30	1.05–1.94	0.02

Aspirin administration

The analysis revealed that patients taking aspirin before admission were more likely to suffer from unstable angina than MI.[15] This is consistent with the hypothesis that aspirin taken before a plaque event attenuates the severity of the response to plaque rupture and the thrombus is, therefore, less likely to be permanent and occlusive. This can be explained by the fact that aspirin irreversibly acetylates platelet cyclo-oxygenase, resulting in the inhibition of thromboxane A_2 synthesis and, thus, platelet activation. It also confirms the findings of others that patients taking aspirin are not only more likely to present with unstable angina than MI, but are also more likely to present with non-Q wave MI than Q wave MI.[16-8] The potential for aspirin to influence the pathogenesis of plaque events in this way may contribute importantly to its well established prognostic benefits in patients with coronary artery disease.[19]

Smoking

Cigarette smoking has prothrombotic effects: it causes increased circulatory levels of fibrinogen and its adverse effects on coronary artery endothelial function have been shown to increase platelet activation and alter secretion of tissue plasminogen activator and its inhibitor, which combine to reduce fibrinolytic activity.[20,21] Such effects increase the probability of coronary occlusion following plaque rupture, suggesting that the adverse prognostic effects of smoking may relate not only to the increased risk of developing atherosclerosis, but also to the increased risk of occlusive thrombus and acute MI.

Increased age

The analysis revealed that the effect of increased age on the mode of presentation of plaque rupture was similar to that of smoking — patients >70 years were shown to be more than twice as likely to have MI than unstable angina. Studies of von Willebrand factor levels and endothelial-dependant vasodilatation indicate that endothelial dysfunction is more prevalent with increasing age.[22] Similarly, levels of fibrinogen and factor VII increase with age, while antithrombin III levels are shown to decrease.[23] Endothelial dysfunction and the imbalance in the coagulation cascade combine to produce a prothrombotic state which may have accounted for this observation — age-related deterioration in renal function, however, may also have contributed.

Renal impairment

Renal impairment, as indicated by increased creatinine levels, was shown to be an independent predictor of presentation with acute MI.[15] This presumably reflects the fact that renal impairment is associated with endothelial dysfunction and a wide range of other abnormalities in the coagulation system, including elevated levels of fibrinogen, increased plasminogen activator inhibitor 1 activity and decreased anti-thrombin III activity.[24,25]

Hypertension

The analysis suggested that hypertensive patients tended to present with unstable angina — this may have been a consequence of left ventricular hypertrophy. The increase in myocardial oxygen demand and the susceptibility to ischaemia would favour presentation with unstable angina in response to minor plaque events that would normally remain silent.

Increased collateralization

The degree of collateralization of the coronary circulation is related to severity and duration of coronary artery disease — patients who have previously been admitted to hospital with unstable angina and MI, and those who have undergone revascularization, may be expected to have more developed collateral circulation.[26] Authors such as Habib *et al* and Christian *et al* have reported that the size of an MI is reduced in individuals with a collateral circulatory supply.[27,28] Thus, it is likely that patients with a history of previous acute coronary syndromes and revascularization procedures were more likely to present with unstable angina as a result of the protective effect of collateral circulation against ischaemic injury following thrombotic coronary occlusion.

Conclusion

Clinical presentation of a plaque rupture is determined by the complex and dynamic interaction of a range of factors, including the nature of the plaque itself and the mechanical and haemodynamic forces acting on it. Our data have shown that factors that influence thrombogenicity, myocardial mass and collateralization of the coronary circulation may also influence the clinical presentation of patients with acute coronary syndromes. Thus, presentation with MI is favoured by cigarette smoking, advanced age and renal impairment, all of which increase thrombogenicity. Presentation with unstable angina is favoured by: treatment with aspirin, which reduces thrombogenicity; hypertension, which increases myocardial mass; and a history of previous coronary syndromes and revascularization procedures which may be associated with increased collateralization of the coronary circulation.

References

1. Buller H, ten Cate J. Coagulation and platelet activation pathways. A review of the key components and the way in which these can be manipulated. *Eur Heart J* 1995; **16**(suppl L): 8–10.
2. Pedersen OD, Gram J, Jespersen J. Plasminogen activator inhibitor type-1 determines plasmin formation in patients with ischaemic heart disease. *Thromb Haemost* 1995; **73**: 835–40.
3. Celermajer DS. Endothelial dysfunction: does it matter? Is it reversible? *J Am Coll Cardiol* 1997; **30**: 325–33.
4. Jaffe E, Hoyer L, Nacman R. Synthesis of von Willebrand factor by cultured human endothelial cells. *Proc Natl Acad Sci* 1987; **79**: 117–23.
5. Rauch U, Chesebro J, Fuster V, Badimon J. Unstable angina and the role of thrombus. *Acute Coron Synd* 1997; **1**: 2–8.
6. Davies MJ, Thomas AC. Plaque fissuring: the cause of acute myocardial infarction, sudden ischaemic death, and crescendo angina. *Br Heart J* 1983; **50**: 127–34.
7. Fuster V, Badimon L, Badimon JJ, Chesebro JH. The pathogenesis of coronary artery disease and the acute coronary syndromes. *N Engl J Med* 1992; **326**: 242–50.
8. Davies MJ, Bland JM, Hangartner JR *et al*. Factors influencing the presence or absence of acute coronary artery thrombi in sudden ischaemic death. *Eur Heart J* 1989; **10**: 203–8.

9. Falk E, Shah PK, Fuster V. Coronary plaque disruption. *Circulation* 1995; **92**: 657–71.

10. Gronholdt M-L, Dalager-Pedersen S, Falk E. Coronary atherosclerosis: determinants of plaque rupture. *Eur Heart J* 1998; **19**: 24–29.

11. Fernandez-Ortiz A, Badimon J, Falk E *et al*. Characterization of the relative thrombogenicity of atherosclerotic plaque components: implications for consequences of plaque rupture. *J Am Coll Cardiol* 1994; **23**: 1562–9.

12. Shiomi M, Ito T, Tsukada T *et al*. Reduction of serum cholesterol levels alters lesional composition of atherosclerotic plaques. Effects of pravastatin sodium on atherosclerosis in mature WHHL rabbits. *Arterioscler Thromb Biol* 1995; **15**: 1938–44.

13. Knoll M, Hellums J, McIntire L *et al*. Platelets and shear stress. *Blood* 1996; **88**: 1525–41.

14. Theroux P, Ouimet H, McCans J *et al*. Aspirin, heparin or both to treat unstable angina. *N Engl J Med* 1988; **319**: 1105–11.

15. Kennon S, Suliman A, MacCallum PK *et al*. Clinical characteristics determining the mode of presentation in patients with acute coronary syndromes. *J Am Coll Cardiol* 1998; **32**: 2018–22.

16. Col NF, Yarzbski J, Gore JM *et al*. Does aspirin consumption affect the presentation or severity of acute myocardial infarction? *Arch Int Med* 1995; **155**: 1386–9.

17. Borzak S, Cannon C, Kraft P *et al*. Effects of prior aspirin and anti-ischemic therapy on outcome of patients with unstable angina. *Am J Cardiol* 1998; **81**: 678–81.

18. Garcia-Dorado D, Theroux P, Tornos P *et al*. Previous aspirin use may attenuate the severity of the manifestation of acute ischemic syndromes. *Circulation* 1995; **92**: 1743–8.

19. Antiplatelet Trialists' Collaboration. Collaborative overview of randomized trials of antiplatelet therapy: Prevention of death, myocardial infarction, and stroke by prolonged antiplatelet therapy in various categories of patients. *BMJ* 1994; **308**: 81–106.

20. Lowe GD, Fowkes FG, Dawes J *et al*. Blood viscosity, fibrinogen, and activation of coagulation and leucocytes in peripheral arterial disease and the normal population in the Edinburgh Artery Study. *Circulation* 1993; **87**:1915–20.

21. Simpson AJ, Gray RS, Moore NR, Booth NA. The effects of chronic smoking on the fibrinolytic potential of plasma and platelets. *Br J Haematol* 1997; **97**: 208–13.

22. Aillaud M, Pignol F, Alessi M *et al*. Increase in plasma concentration of plasminogen activator inhibitor, fibrinogen, von Willebrand factor, factor VIII:C and erythrocyte sedimentation rate with age. *Thromb Haemost* 1986; **55**: 330–2.

23. Lowe GDO, Rumley A, Woodward M *et al*. Epidemiology of coagulation factors, inhibitors and activation markers: the Third Glasgow MONICA Survey. *Br J Haematol* 1997; **97**: 775–84.

24. Haaber AB, Eidemake I, Jensen T *et al*. Vascular endothelial cell function and cardiovascular risk factors in patients with chronic renal failure. *J Am Soc Nephrol* 1995; **5**: 1581–4.

25. Ma K, Greene E, Raij L. Cardiovascular risk factors in chronic renal failure and hemodialysis populations. *Am J Kidney Dis* 1992; **6**: 505–13.

26. Sabri M, DiSciasco G, Cowley M *et al*. Coronary collateral recruitment: functional significance and relation to rate of vessel closure. *Am Heart J* 1991; **121**: 876–80.

27. Habib GB, Heibig J, Forman SA *et al*. Influence of collateral vessels on myocardial infarct size in humans: results of phase 1 Thrombolysis in Myocardial Infarction (TIMI) trial. *Circulation* 1991; **83**: 739–46.

28. Christian T, Gibbons R, Clements I *et al*. Estimates of myocardium at risk and collateral flow in acute myocardial infarction using electrocardiographic indexes with comparison to radionuclide and angiographic measures. *J Am Coll Cardiol* 1995; **26**: 388–93.

Diagnosis in the community

Govindaraj Mohan, James Paget Hospital NHS Trust, Norfolk

Many people with coronary atheroma do not have angina either because the atheroma is not causing obstruction or because gradual obstruction has been compensated for by a collateral circulation. As a result, although most people with angina have coronary atheroma, many of the complications of coronary atheroma (including myocardial infarction (MI) and sudden death) occur in people without any previous known anginal history.[1]

In a few patients, angina is not caused by coronary artery disease but by aortic stenosis or hypertrophic cardiomyopathy. Angina can be made worse by anaemia or hyperthyroidism.

Stable angina is the relative term in contrast to unstable angina, where symptoms progressively increase in severity over a short period of time, and an increased risk of complications such as death or MI occurs. Symptom severity is an imperfect guide to the severity of progression of coronary atheroma.[2]

The cardinal symptom of patients with acute coronary syndromes is chest pain that initiates clinical evaluation. The Braunwald classification was introduced to allow identification of subgroups of unstable angina patients at different levels of cardiac risk.[3] This empirically developed classification is based on pain severity and duration as well as pathogenesis of myocardial ischaemia, and has been validated by prospective studies.[4,5]

The US Agency for Healthcare Policy and Research (AHCPR) clinical practice guidelines for the diagnosis and treatment of unstable angina have helped refine the assessment and management of patients with unstable angina.[6]

Presentation of unstable angina

Unstable angina is an acute coronary syndrome caused by the rupturing of athersclerotic plaques. Plaque rupture initiates the formation of platelet activation and aggregation, which results in thrombus formation. In unstable angina, the thrombus is transient or subocclusive, causing a brief lack of oxygen to the myocardium — this leads to severe, suffocating chest pain, characterizing the condition.

The AHCPR guidelines have conveniently grouped patients into three grades of severity (Table 1).[6] Alternatively, presentation of unstable angina can be viewed according to three broad groups of patients with the following:

- new onset angina occurring either at rest or with minimal effort
- marked increase in anginal severity, or a recurrence of severe angina in a patient with pre-existing disease
- anginal symptoms occurring shortly after an acute MI.

The prognosis of unstable angina has improved over the past 30 years with better risk assessment and early management strategies. The incidence of cardiovascular death or MI is 4.7% at seven days.[7] Recognizing that many patients with unstable angina may progress rapidly to MI or death within a few hours of symptom onset is vital in primary care. Even with maximum medical therapy, 10–15% of patients with unstable angina or non-Q wave MI will die or develop further MI, and a further 35–50% will need coronary revascularization.[8–10]

Thus, unstable angina should be considered a medical emergency warranting urgent hospital admission. Using the above data, agreed standards should be benchmarked in primary care. The following classification is suggested, categorized in terms of risk outcomes towards immediate action plans.

13

Table 1 Short-term risk of death or non-fatal MI in patients with unstable angina[6]

High risk — at least one of the following features must be present:	Intermediate risk — no high-risk feature but must at least one of the following:	Low risk — no high-intermediate risk feature but may have any of the following features:
• Prolonged, ongoing (>20 min) rest pain	• Prolonged (>20 mins) rest angina, now resolved with moderate or high likelihood of CAD	• Increased angina frequency, severity or duration
• Pulmonary oedema, most likely related to ischaemia	• Rest angina (>20 min or relieved with rest or sublingual nitroglycerin)	• Angina provoked at a lower threshold
• Angina at rest with dynamic ST changes >1mm	• Nocturnal angina	• New onset angina with onset two weeks or two months before presentation
• Angina with new or worsening mitral regurg murmur	• Angina with dynamic T wave changes	• Normal or unchanged electrocardiogram
• Angina with S3 or new/worsening rales	• New onset CCSC III or IV angina in the past two weeks with moderate or high likelihood of CAD	
• Angina with hypotension	• Pathologic Q waves or resting ST depression <1mm in multiple lead groups (anterior, inferior, lateral)	
	• Age <65 years	

High-risk cases

Diagnosis

Patients presenting with the following symptoms are generally classified as high-risk cases for unstable angina:

- pain similar to that experienced in angina, but occurring at rest
- new onset angina with marked restriction in less than 25–50 yards activity experienced over the past few weeks
- angina of rapidly increasing severity or frequency that is a changing pattern in a previously stable patient
- anginal pain lasting for more than 15 minutes and not relieved by glyceryl trinitrate
- angina after recent infarction.

These presentations should be identified as the greatest risks and treatment should, therefore, be provided as quickly as possible.

Management strategy

The high-risk unstable angina patient needs immediate admission to hospital. Before admission, however, the following therapies should be instituted:

- soluble aspirin, between 75 and 300 mg:[11–3] large-scale studies have shown that the risk of MI or death is significantly reduced with aspirin treatment both immediately and after the event[14] and over longer periods of time.[15,16] In the RISC study, low dose oral aspirin 75 mg per day reduced the risk of MI or death after an episode of unstable angina or non-Q wave MI by 50% at three months.[16] The incidence of death or MI can be as high as 15% within one month of initial presentation of unstable angina and prompt treatment with aspirin and heparin can reduce this figure to as low as 3–4%[11]
- nitrates: these are useful for pain management and acute ischaemia and should initially be given sublingually or as buccal nitrates (Sustac 2.5 mg buccal)
- oxygen: if the patient does not suffer from chronic obstructive pulmonary disease, a high concentration of oxygen should be given in the surgery and in the ambulance journey.

Direct admission to the hospital coronary care unit (and not via the Accident & Emergency department) is essential. Access to this unit should have been established as a system within the area as an agreed interface protocol. This agreement should have been planned, discussed, agreed and owned by primary care, the emergency ambulance service and secondary care. Fast-track, direct admission to coronary care units in suspected acute MI substantially reduces the time to thrombolysis, as the delays caused by assessment in the casualty department are avoided.[17] A similar system should be adopted for admitting unstable angina patients.

Low-risk cases

Diagnosis

All patients with recent onset, exertional angina without high-risk criteria in presentation should be referred for assessment and risk stratification.[18] General practice assessment before referral should include:

- clinical assessment of symptoms
- clinical examination to identify other possible causes of chest pain and other causes of angina, eg anaemia/valve disease
- assessment of coronary risk factors (family history, smoking, diabetes, hypertension)
- a baseline resting 12-lead electrocardiogram
- cholesterol/high density lipoprotein cholesterol levels.

Referral protocols as agreed and owned between primary and secondary care interface could be utilized for management plan.[19]

Fast-track angina clinics

Direct general practice access to a fast-track angina clinic should be made available within the area. These clinics are provided by physicians with special interest and training in cardiology. The following facilities should be available:

- advice from the specialist
- making a comprehensive cardiological evaluation
- exercise electrocardiography to confirm diagnosis and for risk stratification
- other non-invasive techniques for patients not amenable to exercise electrocardiogram (eg myocardial perfusion, imaging or dipyridamole stress test)
- development of an agreed protocol between secondary and tertiary care when cardiac catheterization and coronary angioplasty or bypass surgery is felt to be necessary on the basis of risk stratification at the clinic. A close-working relationship between secondary care and cardiac specialists (tertiary care) is essential. The standardized, agreed criteria for surgical intervention in an outcome based management structure will need to be reviewed and modified according to emerging evidence.[19]

Medical therapy should be started at the consultation in primary care even before referral to the clinic (Table 2) and should consist of:

- low dose aspirin
- sublingual glyceryl trinitrate for symptom control
- β-blockers — these have been shown to reduce mortality when prescribed to patients before or after MI[20,21]
- diltiazem or verapamil — can be used in the absence of left ventricular dysfunction; these are alternatives in patients with chronic obstructive airways disease or asthma, as β-blockers are contraindicated[22]
- calcium antagonists (dihydropyridines) — ie nifedipine, amlodipine, felodipine, nicardipine and nisoldipine. These agents need to be avoided as monotherapy in unstable angina

- statins at evidence-based dosages — these agents should be administered and maintained, aiming for total cholesterol level of < 5 mmol[23]
- additional therapy when considering potassium channel activators, ie nicorandil, which has its main mode of action as a nitric oxide donor and as a vasodilator, reducing pre- and afterload.
- long-acting nitrates — these should be given either as a long-acting, single day therapy or a twice-daily therapy.

Follow-up

Angina patients who do not need further interventional strategies can be followed-up in general practice according to a planned, working model agreed and developed by primary care and the cardiology department of the local area. This strategy would be complemented by setting up cardiac/angina clinics in general practice.

Nurses should be trained to apply evidence-based strategies for managing patients with established diagnosis of ischaemic heart disease and past MI.[24] Regular call and recall systems in general practice could be utilized for follow-up. A protocol which has been agreed between general practitioners and practice nurses running these clinics should be adopted for secondary prevention of ischaemic heart disease. A re-referral criteria to the cardiology department should also be available at this clinic. Continued teaching and monitoring of the follow up-clinics would need to be facilitated by the health educational system run by the local general practitioner tutors.

Table 2 Classes of agents available for background anti-anginal medication[18]

Pharmacological class	Examples	Main mode of action	Contraindications	Comments
β-adrenoceptor antagonist	Propranolol, timolol, atenolol, metoprolol, nadolol, oxprenolol, pindolol, bisoprolol	Attenuates heart rate	Asthma; caution in heat failure, peripheral vascular disease, diabetics	No convincing evidence; differences between agents affect efficacy, but they may affect acceptability
Organic nitrate	Isosorbide mononitrate	NO donor, vascodilator, reduces pre- and afterload		Give once or twice daily to avoid tachphylaxis. Increase dose slowly to avoid headache
Calcium antagonist; dihydropyridine type	Nifedipine, amlodipine, felodipine, nicardipine, nisoldipine	Vasodilator, reduces pre- and after load	Caution in heart failure; avoid as monotherapy in unstable angina	
Calcium antagonist; rate slowing type	Verapamil, diltiazem	Attenuate heart rate increase on exercise; vasodilator, reduce (mainly) afterload	Risk of bradycardia if combined with b-blocker, caution in heart failure	
Potassium channel activator	Nicorandil	NO donor, vasodilator, reduces pre- and afterload		Induces myocardial preconditioning; clinical significance uncertain

NO — nitric oxide

Conclusion

An outcome-based strategy needs to be developed and maintained for the management of unstable angina in the community.

- High-risk cases should immediately be admitted directly to the local cardiac care unit.
- Recent onset, non-high-risk cases should be referred to a direct access fast-track angina clinic for a comprehensive cardiological evaluation, risk stratification and management strategies to be established.
- All coronary heart disease patients should be followed-up to an evidence-based protocol for secondary prevention in general practice.
- Secondary prevention clinics for ischaemic heart disease, run by practice nurses should be instituted, maintained and monitored; systematic methods for identifying patients with cardiovascular disease should be established.
- Patients identified as having cardiovascular disease should have their risk factors for coronary heart disease assessed, receive appropriate lifestyle advice and support, and be helped to continue taking appropriate medication to reduce their risks.
- Continued teaching and monitoring of the follow-up clinics in general practice would need to facilitated by the health educational system run locally by the general practice clinical tutors.

References

1. Kannel WB, Feinleib M. Natural history of angina pectoris in the Framingham study; prognosis and survival. *Am J Cardiol* 1972; **29**: 154–63.
2. Chester MR, Chen L, Tousoulis D *et al*. Differential progression of complex and smooth lesions within the same coronary tree in men with stable coronary artery disease. *J Am Coll Cardiol* 1995; **25**: 837–42.
3. Braunwald E. Unstable angina: a classification. *Circulation* 1989; **80**: 410–4.
4. Miltenburg-van Zul AJ, Simoons ML, Veerhoek RJ, Bossuyt PM. Incidence and follow-up of Braunwald subgroups in unstable angina pectoris. *J Am Coll Cardiol* 1995; **25**: 1286–92.
5. Cannon CP, McCabe CH, Stone PH *et al*. Prospective validation of the Braunwald classification of unstable angina. Results from the Thrombolysis in Myocardial Ischemia (TIMI) III Registry. *Circulation* 1995; **92**: 1–19.
6. Agency for Health Care Policy and Research, National Heart, Lung and Blood Institute. *Unstable angina: diagnosis and management, clinical practice guideline no. 10*. Rockville: US Department of Health and Human Services, Public Health Service, AHCPR, March 1994; publication no. 94–0602.
7. Yusuf S, Flather M, Pogue J *et al*. Variations between countries in invasive cardiac procedures and outcomes in patients with suspected unstable angina or myocardial infarction without initial ST elevation. *Lancet* 1998; **352**: 507–14.
8. Fragmin during instability in coronary artery disease (FRISC) study group. Low-molecular-weight heparin during instability in coronary artery disease. *Lancet* 1996; **347**: 561–8.
9. TIMI IIIB Investigators. Effects of tissue plasminogen activator and a comparison of early invasive and conservative strategies in unstable angina and non-Q wave myocardial infarction. Results of the TIMI IIIB trial. Thrombolysis in myocardial ischemia. *Circulation* 1994; **89**: 1545–56.
10. Klein W, Buchwald A, Hillis SE *et al*. Comparison of low-molecular-weight heparin with unfractionated heparin acutely and with placebo for six weeks in the management of unstable coronary artery disease. *Circulation* 1997; **96**: 61–6.
11. Lewis HD, David JW, Archibald DG *et al*. Protective effects of aspirin against acute myocardial infarction and death in men with unstable angina: results of a Veterans Administration cooperative study. *N Engl J Med* 1983; **309**: 396–403.
12. Cairns JA, Gent M, Singer J *et al*. Aspirin, sulphinpyrazone, or both in unstable angina: results of a Canadian multicenter trial. *N Engl J Med* 1985; **313**: 1369–85.
13. Theroux P, Ouimet H, McCans J *et al*. Aspirin, heparin or both to treat unstable angina. *N Engl J Med* 1988; **319**: 1105–11.
14. Cannon CP. Optimizing the treatment of unstable angina. *J Thromb Thrombol* 1995; **2**: 205–18.
15. Theroux P, Oiumet H, McCans J *et al*. Aspirin, heparin, or both to treat acute unstable angina. *N Engl J Med* 1988; **319**:1105–11.
16. The RISC Group. Risk of myocardial infarction and death during treatment with low dose aspirin and intravenous heparin in men with unstable coronary artery disease. *Lancet* 1990; **336**: 827–30.

17. Burns JMA, Hogg KJ, Rae AP *et al*. Impact of policy of direct admission to a coronary are unit on the use of thrombolytic treatment. *Br Heart J* 1989; **61**: 322–5.

18. Investigation in Management of Stable Angina Revised Guidelines 1998. *Heart* 1999; **81**: 546–55.

19. Mohan G, Grabau WJ. Fast Track Angina Clinic Interface Guidance 1997 — District Guidelines, Personal Communication.

20. The β-blocker Pooling Project Research Group. β-blocker pooling project (BBPP) subgroup findings from randomised trials in post infarction patients. *Eur Heart J* 1988; **9**: 8–16.

21. Nidorf SM, Thompson PL, Jamrozik KD *et al*. Reduced risk of death at 28 days in patients taking β—blocker before admission to hospital with myocardial infarction. *BMJ* 1990; **300**: 71–4.

22. Joint British recommendations on prevention of coronary heart disease in clinical practice. British Cardiac Society December 1998; **80**(suppl 2): S11.

23. Joint British recommendations on prevention of coronary heart disease in clinical practice. Serum Lipid Management. *Heart* 1998; **80**(suppl 2): S8–9.

24. Campbell NC, Ritchie LD, Thain J *et al*. Secondary prevention in coronary heart disease: a randomised trial of nurse led clinics in primary care. *Heart* 1998; **80**: 447–52.

Prognosis of unstable angina

Diana Holdright, The Middlesex Hospital, London

The prognosis of a patient with unstable angina depends on the accuracy of diagnosis, the pattern of symptom development, the extent of coronary artery disease and the presence of comorbid conditions. The remarkable variability of published outcome data in patients with this condition is partly explained by the difficulty in establishing the diagnosis but also by the number of ischaemic syndromes encompassed by the umbrella term 'unstable angina'.[1] Many different descriptions of unstable angina have been used over the years, including impending acute myocardial infarction (in recognition of the high risk of subsequent infarction), crescendo angina and intermediate coronary syndrome. It was not until the early 1970s that the term 'unstable angina' was accepted.[2]

Classification

Early historical studies showed that unstable angina was associated with a significant risk of progression to myocardial infarction (MI) and death. Further information about the natural history of the condition was obtained by placebo-controlled trials in unstable angina. A study by Cairns, for example, showed a 17% incidence of cardiac death or non-fatal MI at two years in the placebo arm, with most events occurring in the first six months.[3] The risks were highest at the time, and shortly after, the diagnosis was established. However, a useful prognosis could only be determined after the adoption of internationally recognized classification systems such as Braunwald's clinical classification[4] and the practice guideline produced in 1994 by the Agency for Health Care Policy and Research and the National Heart, Lung and Blood Institute.[5]

Under Braunwald's diagnostic classification, patients are classified according to:

- severity of pain — new onset/accelerated (I) or at rest, subacute but not within the preceding 48 hours (II), or acute and within 48 hours (III)
- clinical circumstances — secondary (A): conditions that intensify myocardial ischaemia eg anaemia, primary (B): in the absence of extracardiac conditions, and postinfarction (C).

Variant angina and non-Q wave MI (NQWMI) are not within the classification but are grouped under the umbrella term unstable angina. Braunwald's classification assumes symptoms are due to myocardial ischaemia — which is considered one of the most difficult diagnostic problems faced by the admitting physician — and MI has been excluded by electrocardiographic and enzyme criteria, typically retrospectively.

The more accurate and discriminatory the classification system, the worse the prognosis is for this condition. An adverse prognosis is related to the severity of symptoms and the clinical presentation.[6] A simple classification system was recently proposed and tested by Rizik et al.[7] The system was based primarily on clinical presentation at the time of assessment in the emergency room, as follows: Class I, acceleration of previously existing chronic stable angina (IA without new electrocardiogram (ECG) changes, IB with new changes); Class II, exertional angina of new onset without respect to ECG morphology; Class III, new-onset rest angina; Class IV, protracted pain of >20 min duration/episode with persistent abnormalities of subendocardial ischaemia. The system was tested in 1,387 patients fitting these categories and demonstrated a significant increasing trend in cardiac events from Class I to IV, illustrating the clinical usefulness of the classification system. Table 1 summarizes the clinical classification of unstable angina.

Table 1 Clinical classification of unstable angina

Clinical presentation:	Clinical background:	Specific forms:
• Recent onset angina (<60 days) • Crescendo angina • Pain at rest • Prolonged chest pain	• Post-myocardial infarction • Post-percutaneous transluminal coronary angioplasty • Post-coronary artery bypass surgery	• Variant angina • Non-Q wave myocardial infarction

Prognosis

Patients with new onset, severe angina have a better prognosis than those with rest pain. The prognosis of patients with rest pain improves with an increase in the time interval since the last episode of pain. Patients who develop unstable symptoms postinfarction are a high risk group.

New onset angina

Although the very first development of angina is included in most classification systems of unstable angina, it generally occurs at a relatively high workload and has a fairly stable course. The large series from Duke University demonstrated a 16% cardiac event rate at one year compared with a 7% annual event rate in patients with stable angina.[8] These patients generally have less severe and less extensive coronary artery disease and can usually be managed in the same way as stable angina patients. New onset angina also tends to have a better prognosis than acceleration of previously stable angina.[9]

Crescendo angina

Crescendo angina describes an escalation of symptoms with an increase in frequency, duration and/or severity of chest pain and accounts for most patients diagnosed with unstable angina who are at considerable risk of MI and its sequelae. A recent review of 10 representative studies encompassing nearly 2,000 patients was undertaken by Betriu and showed that in-hospital mortality rates ranged from 2% to 8% and that one-year survival was 90%.[10] Patients with a recurrence of chest pain in hospital have significantly worse one-year survival.[11]

Non-Q wave myocardial infarction

There is continuous progression from severe unstable angina (without detectable myocardial damage) to NQWMI (with an enzyme rise but without the development of pathological Q wave), through to Q wave MI. The development of even more sensitive assays of myocardial damage, such as the troponin T and I assays, has blurred the distinction between unstable angina and NQWMI.

Although NQWMI is associated with less myocardial necrosis and a more benign in-hospital course than Q-wave MI, many studies have demonstrated a high event rate in the early months after presentation such that medium-term survival is similar.[12] Patients with NQWMIs have a higher rate of rehospitalization for unstable angina and a greater likelihood of undergoing bypass surgery or coronary angioplasty (Figure 1).[12]

Extension of infarction in patients with NQWMI identifies a subgroup of patients with a poorer prognosis. This was demonstrated in a study carried out by Maisel et al involving 1,253 patients with Q wave and NQWMI.[13] Extension of infarction occurred in 6% and 8% of patients respectively. In these subgroups, in-hospital mortality was 15% in those with Q wave MI and 43% in those with NQWMI ($p<0.01$). One-year survival was similar for both subgroups without extended infarcts (82% vs 84%). Extension of infarction was, therefore, shown to be the strongest univariate predictor of one year mortality in patients with NQWMI.

Early postinfarction angina

Early postinfarction angina describes patients with recurrent chest pain between 24 hours and one month after an acute myocardial infarct. The prevalence of such angina with ECG changes is around 18%, and is more frequent in patients with NQWMI, multivessel disease or previous angina.[14] Survival is lower in this subgroup of patients. Postinfarction angina without ECG changes carries less prognostic significance unless the episodes of pain are frequent ie >1 episode/24 hours.[15]

Gender differences

The difficulties in making a diagnosis of unstable angina in women are well recognized — some women diagnosed with unstable angina are subsequently found to have normal coronary arteries — and explain the better prognosis of women with angina.[16]

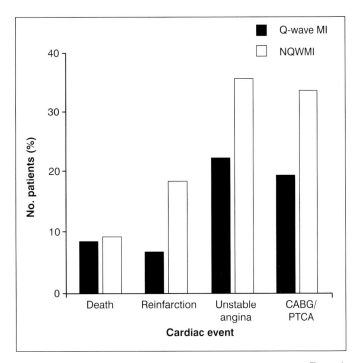

Figure 1: Incidence of cardiac events in Q and non-Q wave MI patients during a 27-month follow-up period[12]

The larger trial of thrombolysis in unstable angina and MI (TIMI IIIB trial) enrolled 497 women and 976 men; for both syndromes, women were older, had a higher frequency of diabetes mellitus and hypertension and were taking more cardiac medications. Although the 42 day death and MI rates were shown to be similar for women and men (7.4% vs 7.5%), coronary angiography revealed less severe disease in women; there was also absence of critical obstructions in 25% of women compared with 16% of men. The similar outcome in men and women suggests that the older age and greater comorbidity of women offset the more favourable angiographic findings. The most important clinical variables predictive of outcome in TIMI IIIB were age and the presence of ST segment depression.[17]

Symptom severity

Traditionally, patients with recurrent and/or severe chest pain are treated more aggressively and are likely to be put forward for angiography. Bugiardini studied 104 patients with unstable angina using symptom diaries, Holter ECG monitoring and angiography within one week of admission; 41 patients had a subsequent coronary event. Anginal scores showed high specificity but low sensitivity for predicting subsequent events. The presence of transient myocardial ischaemia was a better predictor (sensitivity 80% and specificity 89%).[18]

Subjective evaluation of clinical risk has its limitations. This has been demonstrated in Andersen's study. The admitting physicians (internist or cardiologist) were asked to classify 195 patients admitted with unstable angina according to the perceived risk of an adverse clinical outcome, using whatever clinical, ECG or other information were available at that time. Although the clinical risk evaluation was useful for identifying a subgroup of low risk patients during a one year follow-up, it was less effective at identifying high risk groups. Overall, the association between the perceived risk on admission and the final outcome was not strong.[19]

Objective predictors of prognosis

Determining whether chest pain is myocardial in origin can be notoriously difficult and many adjuncts are used to help make a diagnosis. Factors used to risk stratify patients include ECG changes (including the type and extent), blood tests (cardiac enzymes including troponins T and I), extent of myocardium at risk (from ECG, nuclear, echo, and angiographic data) and comorbid conditions.

Resting 12-lead ECG

Ischaemic ST segment changes on the resting ECG identify a group of patients with an adverse prognosis.[20] The TIMI III registry database indicated that patients with ST segment deviation experienced a one year incidence of death or MI of 11%, compared with 8.2% in patients with no ECG changes.[21] T wave changes in isolation were not predictive, with a one year event rate of 6.8%. Patients with left bundle branch block had the highest one year event rate (22.9%).

Recurrent ischaemia in hospital occurred more frequently in patients with ST segment deviation at presentation (19%), compared with 11% in patients with T wave changes on admission and 7.5% in patients without admission ECG changes. Among patients with ST segment changes on admission, anterior changes carried the worst prognosis with a rate of death or MI at one year of 12.4%, compared with 7–8% for other locations or no ST segment deviation. The TIMI registry also found that ST segment deviation of 0.5 mm was as useful a prognostic indicator as ≥1 mm ST segment deviation.

Continuous ST segment monitoring

Continuous recording of the ECG gives more prognostic information than isolated 12-lead ECGs. The detection of episodes of ischaemia, silent or otherwise, in patients hospitalized for unstable angina identifies a subgroup at increased risk of further cardiac events (Figure 2).[22-6] In a study of 212 patients with unstable angina followed for a mean of 2.6 years, admission ECG ST depression and the presence of transient myocardial ischaemia predicted increased risk of death or MI, whereas a normal admission ECG carried a good prognosis.[22] In 14 patients, ST segment monitoring provided the only evidence of recurrent ischaemia, and 72% of this group suffered an adverse event. Transient ischaemia and a history of hypertension were the most powerful independent predictors of death and MI.

In a prospective study of 135 patients with unstable angina, Langer *et al* showed that ST shift on the admission ECG was associated with an unfavourable in-hospital outcome (55% vs 25% in patients without ST shift), with multivessel disease (77% vs 63%), and left main stem disease (22% vs 7%).[27] Comparing patients with and without ST shift on Holter monitoring, an unfavourable outcome was found in 48% vs 20% respectively, multivessel disease in 76% vs 54% and left main stem disease in

Figure 2: Survival rates from MI and death in the presence (TMI +ve) and absence (TMI -ve) of myocardial ischaemia on Holter monitoring[26]

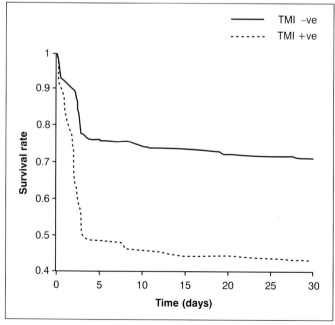

18% vs 4%. Ninety-two per cent of episode of ST shift were asymptomatic and would not, therefore, have been otherwise detected. ST segment shift on Holter monitoring not only predicts an adverse in-hospital prognosis but is also associated with a poorer prognosis in the medium-term.[28]

The association of an adverse prognosis in the presence of transient myocardial ischaemia has been shown in numerous studies in recent years but has not entered routine clinical practice, mainly because it requires off-line analysis, a skilled cardiac technician, is time-consuming and does not provide an instantaneous result. Continuous, on-line vectorcardiography has been developed in an attempt to circumvent some of these issues and may become more widely accepted in the future.[29]

Coronary lesion morphology and transient myocardial ischaemia

The relationship between coronary lesion morphology and transient ischaemia was demonstrated by Pozzati.[30] Patients admitted with unstable angina underwent Holter monitoring during the first 2–4 days, while receiving intensive medical therapy. Coronary angiography was performed within 12 days of admission which showed transient myocardial ischaemia to be greatest in patients with complex coronary morphology (85 +/– 60 mins/24 hour) than in those with regular, smooth morphology or coronary spasm (33 +/– 26 mins/24 hour, $p<0.005$). Medical treatment reduced, but did not abolish, myocardial ischaemia in all groups. The presence of complex coronary morphology or transient myocardial ischaemia were both predictive of in-hospital outcome. Following discharge, persistence of myocardial ischaemia correlated with clinical outcome — lesion morphology did not.

Cardiac troponins

The classical serum marker of cardiac muscle injury, creatine kinase, and its MB isoenzyme creatine kinase-MB, suffer from a lack of specificity and sufficient sensitivity to detect small amounts of myocardial injury. As a result, immunoassays have been developed in recent years to measure serum levels of cardiac troponin I and T, two proteins that regulate myosin-actin interactions. Since the amino acid sequences of these cardiac troponins differ from their skeletal muscle counterparts, assays with minimal cross-reactivity could be developed. Several large studies have recently demonstrated the prognostic value of a single measurement of cardiac troponins in patients with acute ischaemic syndromes.[31–3] The prognostic value of troponin T measured shortly after admission extends beyond the in-hospital phase. In a study by Stubbs, the increased risk associated with a positive assay extended to two years after first presentation.[34] The combination of troponin T measurement and pre-discharge exercise tests is particularly useful as a prognostic indicator.[35]

Other serum markers

Recent work has highlighted the role of inflammation in the acute ischaemic syndromes. Raised levels of the acute phase reactants, such as plasma C-reactive protein, serum amyloid[36] and fibrinogen,[37] predict a worse outcome in patients with unstable angina. Similarly, an association has been found between increased plasma viscosity and erythrocyte aggregation and an unfavourable outcome[38] and between plasma fibrinopeptide amyloid levels, a marker of thrombin activity, and outcome.[39]

Predischarge exercise testing

The prognostic value of a predischarge exercise test has been shown in many studies, predominantly in men but also more recently in women.[40] Due to increased incidence of cardiac events in the weeks after discharge, the test should be performed prior to discharge, and can be carried out safely.[41] The inability to perform a predischarge exercise test is indicative of an adverse prognosis.[42]

The extent and severity of ischaemic change and low peak workload are indicative of a poor prognosis.[35,43] In the RISC study of unstable angina, patients with ST depression on

23

exercise testing had a higher rate of MI or death at one year (18%) compared with those without ST depression (9%, $p<0.01$).[44] This increased risk was not influenced by the presence or absence of pain on the exercise test. However, ST depression combined with pain predicted development of angina at follow-up.

Nuclear perfusion imaging

Perfusion imaging of the heart using thallium or technetium tracers delineates the extent of fixed and reversible perfusion defects, which correlate with the risk of future cardiac events.[45] The technique is particularly useful in patients unable to perform conventional treadmill or bicycle exercise and in those with an abnormal resting ECG. In a recent study of the value of predischarge dipyridamole technetium 99m sestamibi myocardial tomography in medically treated patients with unstable angina, an abnormal scan was present in 77% of patients.[46] A cardiac event occurred in 10% of patients with a normal MIBI result compared with 69% patients with an abnormal result.

Stress echocardiography

This is a more recently developed technique for detecting inducible myocardial ischaemia. It is a useful alternative to nuclear perfusion imaging.

Angiography

Angiographic predictors of an adverse prognosis relate particularly to the extent and severity of coronary artery disease and to left ventricular function. In addition, complex plaque morphology and the presence of intracoronary thrombus are predictive of future cardiac events.[30,47] Although it may identify high-risk patients, routine coronary angiography followed by revascularization has not been shown in large-scale trials to be associated with a better prognosis compared with conservative treatment.[48,49] This procedure should therefore be reserved for patients with spontaneous or inducible ischaemia despite medical therapy and for other high risk patients.

In the UK, whether or not a patient with unstable angina is seen by a cardiologist depends on the local healthcare system and the practice of the admitting physician. A recent study from the US to determine whether or not the outcome of patients with unstable angina was affected by the specialty of the attending physician showed that the mortality rate was higher in the internist group, although it did not achieve statistical significance.[50] With our current healthcare system it is not possible, and some might argue it unnecessary, for all patients with unstable angina to be cared for by or have shared care from a cardiologist.

Conclusion

Diagnosis of unstable angina can be difficult and getting it right and wrong both carry considerable significance for the patient. Classification systems and many objective predictors help improve the accuracy of diagnosis and plan appropriate treatment. However, the very nature of the condition lends itself to treatment guidelines which could ensure that the best possible care is delivered to these patients, irrespective of the specialty of the attending physician.

References

1. Theroux P, Lidon R-M. Unstable angina: pathogenesis, diagnosis, and treatment. *Curr Probl Cardiol* 1993; **18**: 157–232.
2. Fowler NO. 'Preinfarction' angina: a need for an objective definition and for a controlled clinical trial of its management. *Circulation* 1971; **44**: 755–8.
3. Cairns JA, Gent M, Singer J *et al*. Aspirin, sulfinpyrazone, or both in unstable angina. *N Engl J Med* 1985; **22**: 1369–75.

4. Braunwald E. Unstable angina. A Classification. *Circulation* 1989; **80**: 410–4.

5. Braunwald E, Jones RH, Mark DB *et al*. Diagnosing and managing unstable angina. *Circulation* 1994; **90**: 613–22.

6. Theroux P. A pathophysiological basis for the clinical classification and management of unstable angina. *Circulation* 1987; **75**(suppl V): V103–9.

7. Rizik DG, Healy S, Margulis A *et al*. A new clinical classification for hospital prognosis of unstable angina pectoris. *Am J Cardiol* 1995; **75**: 993–7.

8. Roberts KB, Califf RM, Harrell FE *et al*. The prognosis for patients with new onset angina who have undergone cardiac catheterisation. *Circulation* 1983; **68**: 970–8.

9. White LD, Lee TH, Cook EF *et al*. Comparison of the natural history of new onset and exacerbated chronic ischaemic heart disease. *J Am Coll Cardiol* 1990; **16**: 304–10.

10. Betriu A, Heras M, Cohen M, Fuster V. Unstable angina: outcome according to clinical presentation. *J Am Coll Cardiol* 1992; **19**: 1659–63.

11. Gazes PC, Mobley EM, Faris HM *et al*. Preinfarction (unstable) angina—a prospective study—ten year follow-up. *Circulation* 1973; **48**: 331–7.

12. Gibson RS. Clinical, functional, and angiographic distinctions between Q wave and non-Q wave myocardial infarction: evidence of spontaneous reperfusion and implications for intervention trials. *Circulation* 1987; **75**(suppl V): V128–38.

13. Maisel AS, Ahnve S, Gilpin E *et al*. Prognosis after extension of myocardial infarct: the role of Q wave or non-Q wave infarction. *Circulation* 1985; **71**: 211–7.

14. Bosch X, Theroux P, Waters DD *et al*. Early postinfarction ischemia: clinical, angiographic, and prognostic significance. *Circulation* 1987; **75**: 988–95.

15. Benhorin J, Nadrews ML, Carleen ED, Moss AJ, Multicenter Postinfarction Research Group. Occurrence, characteristics and prognostic significance of early postacute myocardial infarction angina pectoris. *Am J Cardiol* 1988; **62**: 679–85.

16. Murabito JM, Evans JC, Larson MG, Levy D. Prognosis after the onset of coronary heart disease. An investigation of differences in outcome between the sexes according to initial coronary disease presentation. *Circulation* 1993; **88**: 2546–55.

17. Hochman JS, McCabe CH, Stone PH *et al*. Outcome and profile of women and men presenting with acute coronary syndromes: a report from TIMI IIIB. *J Am Coll Cardiol* 1997; **30**: 141–8.

18. Bugiardini R, Borghi A, Pozzati A et al. Relation of severity of symptoms to transient myocardial ischemia and prognosis in unstable angina. *J Am Coll Cardiol* 1995; **25**: 597–604.

19. Andersen K, Eriksson P, Dellborg M. Non-invasive risk stratification within 48h of hospital admission in patients with unstable coronary disease. *Eur Heart J* 1997; **18**: 780–8.

20. Patel DJ, Holdright DR, Knight CJ *et al*. Early continuous ST segment monitoring in unstable angina: prognostic value additional to the clinical characteristics and the admission electrocardiogram. *Heart* 1996; **75**: 222–8.

21. Cannon CP, McCabe CH, Stone PH *et al*. The electrocardiogram predicts one-year outcome of patients with unstable angina and non-Q wave myocardial infarction: results of the TIMI III registry ECG ancillary study. *J Am Coll Cardiol* 1997; **30**: 133–40.

22. Patel DJ, Knight CJ, Holdright DR *et al*. Long-term prognosis in unstable angina. The importance of early risk stratification using continuous ST segment monitoring. *Eur Heart J* 1998; **19**: 240–9.

23. Johnson SM, Mauritson DR, Winniford MD et al. Continuous electro-cardiographic monitoring in patients with unstable angina pectoris: identification of high-risk subgroup with severe coronary disease, variant angina, and/or impaired early prognosis. *Am Heart J* 1982; **103**: 4–12.

24. Gottlieb SO, Weisfeldt ML, Ouyang P *et al*. Silent ischemia as a marker for early unfavorable outcomes in patients with unstable angina. *N Engl J Med* 1986; **314**: 1214–9.

25. Nadamanee K, Intarachot V, Josephson MA *et al*. Prognostic significance of silent myocardial ischemia in patients with unstable angina. *J Am Coll Cardiol* 1987; **10**: 1–9.

26. Holdright D, Patel D, Cunningham D *et al*. Comparison of the effect of heparin and aspirin versus aspirin alone on transient myocardial ischemia and in-hospital prognosis in patients with unstable angina. *J Am Coll Cardiol* 1994; **24**: 39–45.

27. Langer A, Freeman MR, Armstrong PW. ST segment shift in unstable angina: pathophysiology and association with coronary anatomy and hospital outcome. *J Am Coll Cardiol* 1989; **13**: 1495–1502.

28. Gottleib SO, Weisfeldt ML, Ouyang P et al. Silent ischemia predicts infarction and death during 2 year follow-up of unstable angina. *J Am Coll Cardiol* 1987; **10**: 756–60.

29. Andersen K, Eriksson P, Dellborg M. Ischaemia detected by continuous on-line vectorcardiographic monitoring predicts unfavourable outcome in patients admitted with probable unstable coronary disease. *Coron Artery Dis* 1996; **7**: 753–60.

30. Pozzati A, Bugiardini R, Borghi A *et al*. Transient ischaemia refractory to conventional medical treatment in unstable angina: angiographic correlates and prognostic implications. *Eur Heart J* 1992; **13**: 360–5.

31. Ohman EM *et al* for the GUSTO-IIa investigators. Cardiac troponin T levels for risk stratification in acute myocardial ischemia. *N Engl J Med* 1996; **335**: 1333–41.

32. Antman EM, Tanasijevic MJ, Thompson B *et al*. Cardiac-specific troponin I levels to predict the risk of mortality in patients with acute coronary syndromes. *N Engl J Med* 1996; **335**: 1342–9.

33. Lindahl B, Venge P, Wallentin L. Relation between troponin T and the risk of subsequent cardiac events in unstable coronary disease. *Circulation* 1996; **93**: 1651–7.

34. Stubbs P, Collinson P, Moseley D et al. Prospective study of the role of cardiac troponin T in patients admitted with unstable angina. *BMJ* 1996; **313**: 262–4.

35. Lindahl B, Andren B, Ohlsson J *et al* and the RISK study group. Risk stratification in unstable coronary artery disease. Additive value of troponin T determinations and pre-discharge exercise test. *Eur Heart J* 1997; **18**: 762–70.

36. Liuzzo G, Biasucci LM, Gallimore R *et al*. The prognostic value of C-reactive protein and serum amyloid A protein in severe unstable angina. *N Engl J Med* 1994; **331**: 417–24.

37. Becker RC, Cannon CP, Bovill E *et al*. Prognostic value of plasma fibrinogen concentration in patients with unstable angina and non-Q-wave myocardial infarction (TIMI IIIB Trial). *Am J Cardiol* 1996; **78**: 142–7.

38. Neumann F-J, Katus HA, Hoberg E *et al*. Increased plasma viscosity and erythrocyte aggregation: indicators of an unfavourable clinical outcome in patients with unstable angina pectoris. *Br Heart J* 1991; **66**: 425–30.

39. Ardissino D, Merlini PA, Gamba G *et al*. Thrombin activity and early outcome in unstable angina pectoris. *Circulation* 1996; **93**: 1634–9.

40. Safstrom K, Nielsen NE, Bjorkholm A *et al* and the IRIS study group. Unstable coronary artery disease in post-menopausal women. Identifiying patients with significant coronary artery disease by basic clinical parameters and exercise test. *Eur Heart J* 1998; **19**: 899–907.

41. Swahn E, Areksog M, Wallentin L. Early exercise testing after coronary care for suspected unstable coronary artery disease—safety and diagnostic value. *Eur Heart J* 1986; **7**: 594–601.

42. Krone RJ, Gregory JJ, Freedland KE. Limited usefulness of exercise testing and thallium scintigraphy in evaluation of ambulatory patients several months after recovery from an acute coronary event: implications for management of stable coronary heart disease. Multicenter Myocardial Ischemia Research Group. *J Am Coll Cardiol* 1994; **24**: 1274–81.

43. Nyman I, Wallentin L, Areksog M *et al* and the RISC Study Group. Risk stratification by early exercise testing after an episode of unstable coronary artery disease. *Int J Cardiol* 1993; **39**: 131–42.

44. Nyman I, Larsson H, Areksog M *et al* and the RISC Study Group. The predictive value of silent ischaemia at an exercise test before discharge after an episode of unstable coronary artery disease. *Am Heart J* 1992; **123**: 324–31.

45. Marmur JD, Freeman MR, Langer A, Armstrong PW. Prognosis in medically stabilised unstable angina: early Holter ST-segment monitoring compared with predischarge exercise thallium tomography. *Ann Intern Med* 1990; **113**: 575–9.

46. Stratmann HG, Tamesis BR, Younis LT *et al*. Prognostic value of predischarge dipyridamole technetium 99m sestamibi myocardial tomography in medically treated patients with unstable angina. *Am Heart J* 1995; **130**: 734–40.

47. Freeman MR, Williams AE, Chisholm RJ, Armstrong PW. Intracoronary thrombus and complex morphology in unstable angina. Relation to timing of angiography and in-hospital cardiac events. *Circulation* 1989; **80**: 17–23.

48. Boden WE, O'Rourke RA, Crawford MH *et al*. Outcomes in patients with acute non-Q wave myocardial infarction randomly assigned to an invasive as compared with a conservative management strategy. *N Engl J Med* 1998; **338**: 1785–92.

49. Anderson HV, Cannon CP, Stone PH *et al*. One year results of the Thrombolysis in Myocardial Infarction (TIMI) IIIB clinical trial: a randomised comparison of tissue-type plasminogen activator versus placebo and early invasive versus early conservative strategies in unstable angina and non-Q wave myocardial infarction. *J Am Coll Cardiol* 1995; **26**: 1643–50.

50. Schreiber TL, Elkhatib A, Grines CL, O'Neill WW. Cardiologist versus internists management of patients with unstable angina: treatment patterns and outcomes. *J Am Coll Cardiol* 1995; **26**: 577–82.

Medical treatment of unstable angina

Robert Henderson, Cardiology Department, Nottingham City Hospital, Nottingham

Myocardial infarction (MI) and unstable angina are both acute coronary syndromes. The pathophysiology of these conditions has not been fully elucidated, but evidence from basic and clinical studies suggests that most cases are caused by disruption of vulnerable atherosclerotic plaques. Such plaques are characterized by reduced smooth muscle content and a thin fibrous cap overlying a large, extracellular, lipid core. Evidence suggests that the fibrous cap is weakened by inflammatory processes and release of enzymes from macrophages, which degrade connective tissue matrix proteins.[1–3] Rupture of the fibrous cap exposes sub-intimal tissues and the lipid-rich core to circulating blood, which stimulates platelet aggregation and activation of the coagulation cascade. An intracoronary thrombus is consequently formed and this can obstruct coronary blood flow and lead to myocardial ischaemia. Knowledge that platelets and the coagulation cascade both play a role in the pathogenesis of acute coronary syndromes has increased research interest in the therapeutic potential of antiplatelet and anti-thrombin agents.

Patients with unstable angina and non-Q wave MI are at risk of adverse cardiac events.[4] Medical treatment aims to stabilize the clinical syndrome, prevent progression to MI and reduce cardiovascular risk. Most patients are admitted to hospital for bed rest and are treated with anti-ischaemic, antiplatelet and anti-thrombin agents. Although there is limited evidence to suggest that hospital admission alone influences clinical outcome, the efficacy of these medical treatment strategies has been confirmed in several clinical trials.

Anti-ischaemic agents

Anti-ischaemic medication, including β-blockers, nitrate preparations and calcium channel blockers, is widely used to relieve symptoms and prevent recurrence of ischaemia in patients with unstable angina. Several trials have demonstrated that β-blockers reduce the frequency and duration of ischaemic episodes in unstable angina patients, but these have been too small to provide definitive information about the effect of β-blockers on prognosis.[5] A meta-analysis of 4,700 patients with ischaemic chest pain and either ST segment depression or a normal electrocardiogram (a condition known as 'threatened MI') suggested that β-blockers reduce the risk of progression to MI by 13%.[6]

There is no evidence that short- and long-acting nitrate preparations and calcium antagonists decrease the risk of major cardiac events in patients with unstable angina.[7] Moreover, dihydropyridine calcium channel antagonists cause reflex tachycardia and can increase myocardial oxygen demand — one trial associated nifedipine with an increased risk of adverse events.[5] Dihydropyridines should, therefore, only be prescribed in combination with a β-blocker. Heart rate-limiting calcium channel blockers, such as diltiazem, may be useful, particularly if β-blockade is contraindicated.[8]

Antiplatelet agents

Aspirin

Several randomized clinical trials have demonstrated that aspirin (in daily doses ranging from 75 mg to 1,300 mg) reduces the risk of death and MI in patients with unstable angina. These results have been confirmed by a meta-analysis involving more than 4,000 unstable angina patients, in which antiplatelet therapy (mainly aspirin) reduced the relative risk of MI, stroke or vascular death by about 40%.[9] It is, therefore, recommended that all patients with acute coronary syndromes be treated with aspirin; although the optimal dose remains unknown, an initial dose of 150–300 mg will provide a rapid antiplatelet effect with a low incidence of gastrointestinal side-effects. In the longer term, a dose of 75 mg daily has been shown to be well tolerated and is effective in patients with stable coronary artery disease.[10]

Thienopyridines

Thienopyridines, such as ticlopidine and clopidogrel, inhibit platelet aggregation induced by adenosine diphosphate. The role of these agents in clinical practice remains uncertain. In one randomized trial involving 652 patients with unstable angina, ticlopidine reduced the six-month risk of vascular death or non-fatal MI from 13.6% to 7.3%, but none of the patients were given aspirin or heparin.[11] Ticlopidine was, however, associated with gastrointestinal side-effects and skin reactions (in 5.1% and 1.9% of patients respectively) and, in other studies, has been shown to cause bone marrow toxicity. Clopidogrel is associated with fewer side-effects and may be an alternative to aspirin for secondary prophylaxis in patients with vascular disease.[12]

Glycoprotein IIb/IIIa receptor antagonists

Over the past few years, the central role of the platelet glycoprotein IIb/IIIa receptor in platelet aggregation has been elucidated. Several new antiplatelet agents that block this receptor and inhibit platelet aggregation have been developed, including abciximab (a chimeric antibody fragment), eptifibatide (a cyclic heptapeptide) and tirofiban and lamifiban (non-peptide molecules). Abciximab, eptifibatide and tirofiban are in clinical use.

Randomized placebo controlled trials have assessed the effect of these receptor antagonists in patients undergoing percutaneous coronary intervention. These studies randomized more than 14,000 patients and demonstrated that glycoprotein IIb/IIIa receptor inhibition reduces 30-day risk of death or MI by about 35%.[13-8] Long-term follow-up of these trials is limited but, in the EPIC study, three-year mortality in patients with unstable angina and evolving MI was 5.1% in patients treated with abciximab and 12.7% in those treated with placebo.[13]

Routine glycoprotein IIb/IIIa blockade in patients with acute coronary syndromes without persistent ST elevation also reduces the risk of adverse cardiac events. In four trials involving more than 16,000 patients, treatment with a glycoprotein IIb/IIIa receptor antagonist reduced the 30-day risk of death or non-fatal MI by 11% — this benefit was particularly marked among patients undergoing percutaneous coronary intervention.[19-22]

The effect of glycoprotein IIb/IIIa inhibitors on the requirement for revascularization has also been reported in several clinical trials. Treatment with these antagonists during percutaneous coronary intervention reduces the need for urgent stent placement, although the need for repeat revascularization procedures has not been reduced consistently.[23] Similar results have been reported in patients with unstable angina. In the PURSUIT trial, more than 59% of patients treated with eptifibatide or placebo underwent coronary arteriography and, at 30 days, no difference in the use of revascularization procedures was shown between the two arms.[22]

Adverse effects

The main adverse effect of glycoprotein IIb/IIIa receptor antagonists is haemorrhage from vascular access sites; early removal of the arterial sheath combined with the use of low-dose heparin has been shown to reduce this risk.[15,24] These inhibitors also increase the risk of haemorrhage during coronary artery bypass surgery, but intracranial and other serious spontaneous haemorrhage rarely occur.[25]

Thrombocytopenia, which can be severe and may require platelet transfusion, is another risk.[26,27] Some patients given abciximab may also develop antibodies to the murine component of the monoclonal antibody,[27] but the clinical significance of this immunological reaction is uncertain.

Glycoprotein IIb/IIIa receptor antagonists are expensive and information about cost and cost-effectiveness is limited. These agents are, therefore, unlikely to be used routinely in all patients with unstable coronary syndromes. Recent evidence suggests that the benefit of glycoprotein IIb/IIIa receptor blockade in acute coronary syndromes is greatest among patients undergoing percutaneous coronary intervention and patients with raised serum troponin levels, and risk stratification may increase clinical and cost-effectiveness.[28]

Anti-thrombin agents

Unfractionated heparin

Unfractionated heparin has been a standard treatment for unstable angina for several years, and clinical practice guidelines advocate intravenous heparin for patients with unstable angina judged to be at intermediate- or high-risk of adverse cardiac events.[29] Evidence to support the use of unfractionated heparin in patients with unstable angina, however, is limited to several small, randomized clinical trials that lack statistical power to detect major clinical outcome differences. In a meta-analysis of six trials including 1,353 patients with unstable angina, the incidence of death or MI during treatment with unfractionated heparin and aspirin was 7.9%, compared with 10.4% with aspirin alone — this difference is of borderline statistical significance.[30]

Unfractionated heparin has a short duration of action and binds extensively to plasma proteins, with unpredictable bioavailability and a variable anticoagulant effect. Unfractionated heparin cannot inhibit thrombin already bound to the thrombus; after cessation of intravenous heparin there may be a rebound increase in thrombin activity, which may be of clinical importance.[31] Heparin is inactivated by platelet factor IV and in some patients heparin causes thrombocytopenia and osteoporosis.[32] These disadvantages of unfractionated heparin have prompted a search for alternative anti-thrombin agents.

Low molecular weight heparins

Low molecular weight heparins, such as dalteparin and enoxaparin, are formed by controlled enzymatic and chemical modification of unfractionated heparin, and act mainly by inhibition of thrombin factors IIa and Xa.[33] The ratio of anti-Xa to anti-IIa activity varies between different low molecular weight heparin preparations and this may account for the differences observed in clinical effect. Low molecular weight heparins offer potential advantages over standard heparin, including a longer duration of action, more predictable bioavailability and anticoagulant effect, and less risk of haemorrhage and thrombocytopenia.[34]

Several recent randomized clinical trials have assessed the use of low molecular weight heparins in patients with unstable angina. In the FRISC trial, for example, 1,506 patients with unstable coronary disease were randomized to either subcutaneous dalteparin or placebo injections. Patients assigned to dalteparin received 120 IU/kg body weight twice daily for six days followed by 7,500 IU once daily for the next 35–45 days. After 40 days, the rate of death and new MI was lower in the dalteparin group than in the placebo group (8.0% versus 10.7%), but this difference attenuated slightly once treatment with dalteparin was discontinued. Dalteparin also reduced the rate of death, new MI or revascularization for incapacitating angina in the long-term, but was associated with an excess of minor bleeds (Figure 1).[35]

The FRIC trial randomized 1,482 patients with unstable angina or non-Q wave MI to the same dose of dalteparin or to unfractionated heparin.[36] During the first six days of the trial, the risk of death, MI and recurrent angina was 9.3% in the dalteparin group and 7.8% in the standard heparin treatment group. Outcome between six and 45 days was the same in both groups, apart from a small excess of minor bleeds in the dalteparin group.

The ESSENCE trial compared subcutaneous enoxaparin (1 mg/kg body weight for 2–8 days) with intravenous unfractionated heparin in 3,171 patients with unstable angina and non-Q wave MI. After 30 days, the rate of death, MI or recurrent angina was significantly lower in the enoxaparin group than in the unfractionated heparin group (19.8% versus 23.3%) (Figure 2).

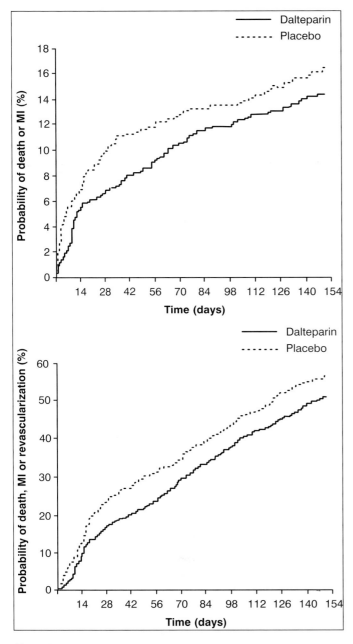

Figure 1:
Cardiac events
in the FRISC trial
after 154 days.

Redrawn and
reproduced with
permission[35]

In addition, the rate of revascularization procedures at 30 days was lower in the enoxaparin group (27.0% versus 32.2%, $p=0.001$), and these differences were maintained over one-year follow-up.[37] Economic analyses suggest that the increased cost of enoxaparin may be compensated by the associated reduction in need for revascularization procedures following treatment,[38] and that routine use of enoxaparin in patients with unstable coronary syndromes may reduce overall costs.

The result of ESSENCE has been confirmed by the TIMI IIB trial, which randomized 3,910 patients with unstable coronary syndromes to enoxaparin or unfractionated heparin. At 14 days, the rate of death, MI or recurrent ischaemia needing revascularization was 14.2% and 16.6% in the enoxaparin and unfractionated heparin groups respectively. This difference was maintained to 43 days but prolonged treatment with a reduced dose of enoxaparin did not confer additional benefit.[39]

Thrombolytic therapy

Several randomized trials have demonstrated that thrombolytic therapy improves angiographic appearance in patients with unstable angina, with less evidence of thrombus and recanalization of some occluded arteries.[40] Thrombolytics do not, however, improve clinical outcome.[41]

Novel anti-thrombins

A range of new, direct thrombin inhibitors is currently being evaluated in patients with acute coronary syndromes.[42] The GUSTO-IIb trial compared recombinant hirudin with unfractionated heparin in 12,142 patients with acute coronary syndromes. Recombinant hirudin was shown to reduce the risk of death or non-fatal MI at 30 days from 9.8% to 8.9%, but was associated with a higher risk of moderate bleeding (8.8% versus 7.7%, $p=0.03$).[43] Similar results have been reported from the OASIS[44] trial. Other direct thrombin inhibitors such as argatroban and efegatran are in the early stages of clinical evaluation.[45]

Future treatments

Greater understanding of the pathophysiology of acute coronary syndromes is needed to enable cardiologists to explore new therapeutic avenues for their patients. Agents currently undergoing evaluation include anti-inflammatory drugs, antibiotics, and novel anti-thrombin and antiplatelet agents.

Conclusion

The optimal medical treatment strategy for patients with unstable angina is still uncertain, but anti-anginal drugs are widely prescribed for symptom-relief. Randomized trial data indicate that treatment with aspirin improves outcome in unstable angina patients, and unfractionated heparin may confer additional benefit. Glycoprotein IIb/IIIa receptor inhibitors are an important new class of antiplatelet agent — they reduce risk in unstable angina patients and in those undergoing percutaneous coronary intervention. These agents, however, are expensive and their role in the routine management of acute coronary syndromes has not been fully evaluated. Low molecular weight heparins offer pharmacokinetic and clinical advantages over unfractionated heparin and represent a significant advance in patient management. A range of novel treatments for patients with acute coronary syndromes is currently in development.

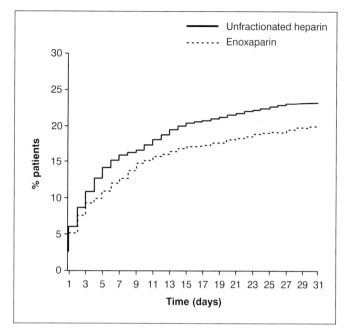

Figure 2: Cardiac events (death, MI or recurrent angina) in the ESSENCE trial.

Redrawn and reproduced with permission[37]

References

1. Libby P. Molecular bases of the acute coronary syndromes. *Circulation* 1995; **91**: 2844–50.

2. Davies MJ. Reactive oxygen species, metalloproteinases, and plaque stability. *Circulation* 1998; **97**: 2382–3.

3. Falk E, Shah PK, Fuster V. Coronary plaque disruption. *Circulation* 1995; **92**: 657–71.

4. Yusuf S, Flather M, Pogue J *et al*. Variations between countries in invasive cardiac procedures and outcomes in patients with suspected unstable angina or myocardial infarction without initial ST elevation. *Lancet* 1998; **352**: 507–14.

5. Holland Interuniversity Nifedipine/Metoprolol Trial. Early treatment of unstable angina in the coronary care unit: a randomized, double-blind, placebo controlled comparison of recurrent ischaemia in patients treated with nifedipine or metoprolol or both. *Br Heart J* 1986; **56**: 400–13.

6. Yusuf S, Wittes J, Friedman L. Overview of results of randomized clinical trials in heart disease. *JAMA* 1988; **260**: 2259–63.

7. Held PH, Yusuf S, Furberg CD. Calcium channel blockers in acute myocardial infarction and unstable angina: an overview. *BMJ* 1989; **299**: 1187–92.

8. Gobel EJ, van Gilst WH, de Kam PJ *et al*. Long-term follow-up after early intervention with intravenous diltiazem or intravenous nitroglycerin for unstable angina pectoris. *Eur Heart J* 1998; **19**: 1208–13.

9. Antiplatelet triallists. Collaborative overview of randomized trials of antiplatelet therapy: prevention of death, myocardial infarction, and stroke by prolonged antiplatelet therapy in various categories of patients. *BMJ* 1994; **308**: 81–106.

10. Juul-Moller S, Edvardsson N, Jahnmatz B *et al*. Double-blind trial of aspirin in primary prevention of myocardial infarction in patients with stable chronic angina pectoris. *Lancet* 1992; **340**: 1421–5.

11. Balsano F, Rizzon P, Violi F *et al*. Antiplatelet treatment with ticlopidine in unstable angina. A controlled multi-center clinical trial. *Circulation* 1990; **82**: 17–26.

12. CAPRIE Steering Committee. A randomized, blinded, trial of clopidogrel versus aspirin in patients at risk of ischaemic events (CAPRIE). *Lancet* 1997; **348**: 1329–39.

13. Topol EJ, Ferguson JJ, Weisman HF *et al*. Long-term protection from myocardial ischemic events in a randomized trial of brief integrin β-3 blockade with percutaneous coronary intervention. *JAMA* 1997; **278**: 479–84.

14. CAPTURE Investigators. Randomized placebo-controlled trial of abciximab before and during coronary intervention in refractory unstable angina: the CAPTURE study. *Lancet* 1997; **349**: 1429–35.

15. EPILOG Investigators. Platelet glycoprotein IIb/IIIa receptor blockade and low-dose heparin during percutaneous coronary revascularization. *N Engl J Med* 1997; **336**: 1689–96.

16. RESTORE Investigators.Randomized Efficacy Study of Tirofiban for Outcomes and REstenosis. Effects of platelet glycoprotein IIb/IIIa blockade with tirofiban on adverse cardiac events in patients with unstable angina or acute myocardial infarction undergoing coronary angioplasty. *Circulation* 1997; **96**: 1445–53.

17. IMPACT-II Investigators. Randomized placebo-controlled trial of effect of eptifibatide on complications of percutaneous coronary intervention: IMPACT-II. *Lancet* 1997; **349**: 1422–8.

18. EPISTENT Investigators. Randomized placebo-controlled and balloon-angioplasty-controlled trial to assess safety of coronary stenting with use of platelet glycoprotein-IIb/IIIa blockade. *Lancet* 1998; **352**: 87–92.

19. PRISM Study Investigators. A comparison of aspirin plus tirofiban with aspirin plus heparin for unstable angina. *N Engl J Med* 1998; **338**: 1498–505.

20. PRISM-PLUS Study Investigators. Inhibition of the platelet glycoprotein IIb/IIIa receptor with tirofiban in unstable angina and non-Q wave myocardial infarction. *N Engl J Med* 1998; **338**: 1488–97.

21. PARAGON Investigators. International, randomized, controlled trial of lamifiban (a platelet glycoprotein IIb/IIIa inhibitor), heparin, or both in unstable angina. *Circulation* 1998; **97**: 2386–95.

22. PURSUIT Trial Investigators. Inhibition of platelet glycoprotein IIb/IIIa with eptifibatide in patients with acute coronary syndromes. Platelet Glycoprotein IIb/IIIa in Unstable Angina: Receptor Suppression Using Integrilin Therapy. *N Engl J Med* 1998; **339**: 436–43.

23. Topol EJ, Serruys PW. Frontiers in interventional cardiology. *Circulation* 1998; **98**: 1802–20.

24. Mandak JS, Blankenship JC, Gardner LH *et al*. Modifiable risk factors for vascular access site complications in the IMPACT II Trial of angioplasty with versus without eptifibatide. Integrilin to Minimize Platelet Aggregation and Coronary Thrombosis. *J Am Coll Cardiol* 1998; **31**: 1518–24.

25. Gammie JS, Zenati M, Kormos RL *et al*. Abciximab and excessive bleeding in patients undergoing emergency cardiac operations. *Ann Thorac Surg* 1998; **65**: 465–9.

26. Berkowitz SD, Harrington RA, Rund MM, Tcheng JE. Acute profound thrombocytopenia after C7E3 Fab (abciximab) therapy. *Circulation* 1997; **95**: 809–13.

27. Ferguson JJ, Kereiakes DJ, Adgey AA *et al*. Safe use of platelet glycoprotein IIb/IIIa inhibitors. *Eur Heart J* 1998; **19**(suppl D): D40–51.

28. Hamm C, Heeschen C, Goldman BU *et al*. Value of throponins in predicting therapeutic efficacy of abciximab in patients with unstable angina. *J Am Coll Cardiol* 1998; **2**: 185A (Abstract).

29. Braunwald E, Jones RH, Mark DB. Diagnosing and managing unstable angina. *Circulation* 1994; **90**: 613–22.

30. Oler A, Whooley MA, Oler J, Grady D. Adding heparin to aspirin reduces the incidence of myocardial infarction and death in patients with unstable angina. *JAMA* 1996; **276**: 811–5.

31. Granger CB, Miller JM, Bovill EG *et al*. Rebound increase in thrombin generation and activity after cessation of intravenous heparin in patients with acute coronary syndromes. *Circulation* 1995; **91**: 1929–35.

32. Hirsh J, Fuster V. Guide to anticoagulant therapy part 1: heparin. *Circulation* 1994; **89**: 1449–68.

33. Weitz JI. Low-molecular-weight heparins. *N Engl J Med* 1997; **337**: 688–98.

34. Siragusa S, Cosmi B, Piovella F *et al*. Low molecular weight heparins and unfractionated heparin in the treatment of patients with acute venous thromboembolism: results of a meta-analysis. *Am J Med* 1996; **100**: 269–77.

35. Fragmin during instability in coronary artery disease (FRISC) Study Group. Low molecular weight heparin during instability in coronary artery disease. *Lancet* 1996; **347**: 561–8.

36. Klein W, Buchwald A, Hillis WS *et al*. Fragmin in unstable angina pectoris or in non-Q wave acute myocardial infarction (the FRIC study). *Am J Cardiol* 1997; **80**: 30E-4E.

37. Cohen M, Demers C, Gurfinkel EP *et al*. A comparison of low molecular weight heparin with unfractionated heparin for unstable coronary artery disease. *N Engl J Med* 1997; **337**: 447–52.

38. Mark DB, Cowper PA, Berkowitz SD *et al*. Economic assessment of low molecular weight heparin (enoxaparin) versus unfractionated heparin in acute coronary syndrome patients: results from the ESSENCE randomized trial. *Circulation* 1998; **97**: 1702–7.

39. Antman EM. Results of TIMI IIB trial. Presented at 20th Congress of European Society of Cardiology, Vienna, 1998.

40. Bar FW, Verheught FW, Col J *et al*. Thrombolysis in patients with unstable angina improves the angiographic outcome but not the clinical outcome. Results of UNASEM, a multicenter, randomized, placebo-controlled, clinical trial with anistreplase. *Circulation* 1992; **86**: 131–7.

41. Anderson HV, Cannon CP, Stone PH *et al*. One-year results of the Thrombolysis in Myocardial Infarction (TIMI) IIIB clinical trial. A randomized comparison of tissue-type plasminogen activator versus placebo and early invasive versus early conservative strategies in unstable angina and non-Q wave myocardial infarction. *J Am Coll Cardiol* 1995; **26**: 1643–50.

42. Lefkovits J, Topol EJ. Direct thrombin inhibitors in cardiovascular medicine. *Circulation* 1994; **90**: 1522–36.

43. The Global Use of Strategies to Open Occluded Coronary Arteries. A comparison of recombinant hirudin with heparin for the treatment of acute coronary syndromes. *N Engl J Med* 1996; **335**: 775–82.

44. OASIS-2 Investigators. Effects of recombinant hirudin (lepirudin) compared with heparin on death, myocardial infarction, refractory angina, and revascularization procedures in patients with acute myocardial ischaemia without ST elevation: a randomized trial. *Lancet* 1999; **353**: 429–38.

45. Simoons M, Lenderink T, Scheffer M *et al*. Efegatran, a new direct thrombin inhibitor: safety and dose response in patients with unstable angina. *Circulation* 1994; **90**: 1–231 (Abstract).

What's really happening in general practice?

John Ferguson, Prescription Pricing Authority, Newcastle-upon-Tyne

Unstable angina is an acute coronary syndrome. Most clinicians use the term 'unstable angina' to denote an accelerating or crescendo pattern of angina, that occurs with less exertion or at rest, lasts longer than stable angina, and is less responsive to medication. Coronary angioscopy has shown that a high proportion of patients with this pattern of symptoms have complex coronary stenoses, characterized by plaque rupture or ulceration, haemorrhage, or thrombosis. This unstable situation may progress to complete occlusion and infarction, or may heal and return to a stable pattern of ischaemia. New-onset angina is sometimes considered unstable but, if it is exertional and responsive to rest and medication, it does not carry the same poor prognosis.

Cardiovascular disease is one of the most common causes of morbidity and mortality. It is the main cause of death in the UK, accounting for around 300,000 deaths/annum. Considerable geographical variation exists with death rates, which are higher in the north of England, urban areas, and areas of social and economic deprivation. Differences in smoking rates and blood pressure levels do not solely explain this variation, and total cholesterol levels do not vary across the country to any great extent. The present preoccupation with cholesterol testing and the availability of lipid-lowering drugs should not prevent us from taking a holistic approach to the patient and to assessing risk factors for cardiovascular disease. Simply treating a laboratory test result should be avoided and the patient's absolute risk of a significant coronary heart disease (CHD) event must be considered.

The National Health Service (NHS) Centre for Reviews and Dissemination reminds us in its *Effective Healthcare bulletin* that cholesterol levels are a poor predictor of those who will develop CHD, and that smokers with high blood pressure have three times the risk of dying from this condition than non-smokers with low blood pressure, when both have the same cholesterol levels.[1] As a result of several high profile clinical trials[2,3] and the Department of Health's 'Health of the Nation' targets,[4] management of health risks associated with hyperlipidaemia has increased in importance and the use of lipid lowering agents escalated over the past few years.

Risk factors known to affect CHD include: smoking, inadequate physical activity, raised blood pressure and blood cholesterol levels. These risk factors are well recognized and fall into two classes: fixed factors, which include family history, male sex, age and diabetes mellitus, and modifiable factors, which include smoking, hypertension, obesity, lack of physical exercise and high cholesterol. The intense current interest in lipids has encouraged a one-dimensional approach to coronary risk based on pre-determined total serum cholesterol or low density lipoprotein cholesterol cut-off points. Epidemiological evidence shows that CHD risk is multifactorial and an individual's risk cannot be determined by considering lipid measurements in isolation.[1] The effects, however, are not simply additive and it is the combination of factors, rather than the individual ones, that need to be considered.

We need to encourage healthy lifestyles among our patients as part of general health promotion. Healthy eating, regular exercise, avoiding obesity, and modest alcohol consumption can all help. Older people, with their intrinsically higher risk of CHD, gain more benefit from health promotion programmes than younger adults. Health promotion activities should be integrated with management of those with hypertension and cardiovascular disease. There are a number of medical treatment methods for unstable angina, which will be discussed in this paper.

Medical treatment methods

Nitrates

Nitrates are first-line, anti-ischaemic therapy for unstable angina. The national usage of nitrates has increased by 25% in the past five years. Glyceryl trinitrate usage has remained relatively constant. There has been a small reduction in the use of isosorbide dinitrate, but a substantial increase in the use of isosorbide mononitrate.

The national cost of nitrates is now £60m/annum[5] and the trends in costs are broadly comparable with trends in usage. Glyceryl trinitrate is increasingly being prescribed as sprays and there has been a corresponding reduction in the sublingual tablets over the years and, more recently, in the patches and modified release tablets, which are expensive ways of prescribing glyceryl trinitrate. There has been a recent trend towards premium-priced modified release isosorbide mononitrate tablets. There is currently a sixfold variation in the use of these drugs by health authority.[5]

Aspirin

Intravascular thrombosis plays a prominent role in the pathophysiology of unstable angina and its progression to myocardial infarction. Anti-thrombotic therapy, therefore, plays an important role in the treatment of unstable angina. Aspirin was first discovered to have anti-platelet properties 30 years ago — it acts to reduce thrombosis and prolong bleeding time. Clinical trials suggest that it should be used, unless contraindicated, to reduce cardiovascular morbidity and mortality in high-risk patients, such as those with coronary artery disease, post-myocardial infarction, and some patients with atrial fibrillation. Low-dose aspirin is inexpensive, effective and relatively safe, with national prescribed usage trebling in the past five years.[5] Though traditionally considered in the management of cerebrovascular ischaemia, its use should be considered in patients with severe myocardial ischaemia.

Low molecular weight heparins

The use of low molecular weight heparins in general practice has increased eightfold in the past six years.[5] The market is currently shared equally by enoxaparin, dalteparin sodium and tinzaparin sodium.[5]

β-blockers

β-blockers are part of the initial treatment of unstable angina unless otherwise contraindicated. If the patient has no history or physical findings of heart failure, these agents can usually be given without measurements of left ventricular function. Patients often avoid using these drugs as they believe they cause fatigue and diminish their exercise capacity, thereby reducing the quality of life. Research studies do not tend to support this belief — one large study recently found that the quality of life was improved with atenolol compared with placebo.[6] Over the past five years, the national trends in the usage of β-blockers has remained relatively constant. Atenolol and propranolol are the most frequently prescribed β-blockers. There has been a small reduction in the use of the disproportionately expensive combination products with β-blockers. Over the past five years, the national costs of these agents have fallen from £116m to £80m/annum, mainly due to the reduced cost of generic atenolol. A threefold variation in the use of these drugs by health authority exists.[5]

Calcium-channel blockers

Calcium-channel blockers have not been shown to favourably affect outcome in unstable angina, and they should be used primarily as third-line therapy in patients with continuing symptoms on nitrates and β-blockers or those who are not candidates for these drugs. In the presence of nitrates and without accompanying β-blockers, diltiazem and verapamil are preferred, since nifedipine and the other dihydropyridines are more likely to cause reflex tachycardia or hypotension. Their safety during long-term treatment is less well established — they should, therefore, be considered for hypertension only when thiazides and β-blockers are contraindicated, not tolerated, or fail to control blood pressure.[7] The national usage of calcium-channel blockers has increased by 50% over the past five years, with a trend towards higher doses and modified release preparations. During this time, nifedipine has remained constant and currently represents 50% usage. Amlodipine, which is marketed as a once-a-day therapy, is now the next most widely used product, followed by diltiazem. There is currently a threefold variation in the use of these drugs by health authority.[5] The usage of verapamil has declined. The national cost of calcium-channel blockers has increased by 62% to £216m/annum over the past five years.

Lipid-lowering agents

Lipid-lowering agents are found within section 2.12 of the British National Formulary and fall into several groups.[7] The main agents are statins and fibrates. The less used groups include omega-3 fish oils, nicotinic acid derivatives, anion exchange resins and, recently, an ispaghula preparation.

The Standing Medical Advisory Committee (SMAC) guidelines,[8] published in 1997 with EL(97) 41,[9] have focused attention on the appropriate selection for treatment of patients at risk from CHD. While many authors have questioned the details of the recommendations made in the SMAC report,[10] it is undoubtedly appropriate to target the use of therapeutic agents such as the statins where the most benefit can be achieved.

The SMAC guidelines refer to the Sheffield tables[11] as a means of assessing the risks of CHD due to different combinations of factors. It has been argued that the New Zealand risk tables[12] are easier to use in practice and give a reasonable basis for assessing risks and deciding when to initiate therapy. These also use the ratio of total cholesterol:high density lipoproteins, which may be a more effective means of measuring the risk of CHD than simple cholesterol levels. The SMAC guidelines also suggest an upper age limit of 70 years, mainly due to lack of evidence from trials of benefits to those aged over 70 for primary prevention of CHD.

The British National Formulary reminds us that all lipid-lowering drugs must be combined with strict adherence to diet, maintenance of new ideal body weight and, if appropriate, reduction of blood pressure and cessation of smoking.[7] No major therapeutic decision, such as introducing a particular restrictive diet or lipid-lowering drugs, should be taken as a result of a single cholesterol determination. At least two or three fasting measurements of cholesterol triglycerides and high density lipoprotein cholesterol are necessary for those whom drug therapy is under consideration.

Prescriptions for lipid-lowering agents account for 4.7% of the cardiovascular prescriptions and 17% of their cost. The costs of lipid-lowering drugs are > 3% of the total prescribing costs.[5] It has also been estimated that the total cost of CHD is about 2.5% of the total NHS budget.[13] The number of patient years represented by the prescriptions for statins is 340,000 using the WHO Defined Daily Dose (DDD).[14] If the suggestions given in the SMAC guidelines which give priority to secondary prevention are followed, the additional costs to the NHS will be substantial.

Statins

Although prescribing for most groups of lipid-lowering drugs is static or declining, statin prescribing is increasing rapidly, especially since the end of 1994 when the Scandinavian Simvastatin Survival (4S) study[2] was published and the first West of Scotland Coronary Prevention Study (WOSCOP) report in 1995.[3] Statins now account for more than 75% of usage and 85% of costs of the lipid-lowering agents. The usage has increased nearly eightfold, from four million DDDs/quarter to more than 31 million DDDs/quarter. Over the same period, costs increased similarly from £4m to £34m/quarter.[5]

Simvastatin currently accounts for 70% of all prescriptions for statins, pravastatin for 14% and fluvastatin for 6%. Atorvastatin and cerivastatin are two new agents — atorvastatin already accounts for 7% of prescriptions and appears to be rapidly increasing.[5]

While studies carried out would seem to suggest that most of the effects of the statins may be described as a class act, there is insufficient evidence currently available to assess the clinical significance of the increased effects of atorvastatin on lowering triglycerides nor on its variable effects on HDL.

The WHO DDDs for statins other than simvastatin are probably higher than those typically used in England. For the two newer statins, atorvastatin and cerivastatin, the British National Formulary doses recommended also appear to be higher than is shown in practice by an examination of actual prescriptions.[15] Is it better to treat more patients for a given total cost with a lower dose, such as is typically used at present, or fewer patient with a higher dose which has been proven in trials to be effective? While the various trials have undoubtedly proved the efficacy of statins, the minimum effective dose is less clear.

Considerable variation across health authorities is seen in the usage of statins as measured by DDDs per 1,000 lipid-lowering specific therapeutic group age-sex related prescribing units (STARPUs).[16] The national average is about 340, but the range is between 200 and 725. Furthermore, no apparent correlation exists between CHD mortality rates (1994/5 data) and usage of statins — some areas have high statin usage and low mortality rates while others have low statin usage with high mortality rates. Even if only the population over 65 is examined, the correlation between mortality figures for a health authority and the level of statin usage is minimal.[17] Overall usage is highest in the North West and lowest in the West Midlands. CHD mortality rates are, however, high in the West Midlands. CHD mortality rates are medium to high in most of the North West, which tends to correlate with statin usage. However, some parts of the South West and South East have low mortality rates but high statin usage. It might be argued that the high use of statins was helping prevent CHD. However, the latest mortality data available refers to 1994/5 and the mortality rates in the South West and South East were low then, before the large increase in statin usage in the wake of the 4S and WOSCOP trials.

Geographical variations in the occurrence of CHD as well as the other risk factors discussed above should, therefore, be considered when deciding prescribing policies. In all health authorities, simvastatin is the most commonly used statin, in most pravastatin is the second most common, but in a few atorvastatin already holds that position.[5] In a sample of prescriptions recently dispensed,[15] 53% were for men and 44% for women. The remaining 3% did not specify. It is considered that women are just as likely to suffer from CHD as men, only to suffer it later in life, typically when over 70 and thus, in theory, above the upper age recommended by SMAC. There is currently a 3.6-fold variation in the use of these drugs by health authority.[5]

Fibrates

Clofibrate, the first of this group to be launched, has been on the market for more than 30 years. It is now, however, restricted in its use to those patients who have had a cholecystectomy and its use is declining. Other fibrates have more recently been introduced. Bezafibrate remains the most commonly used agent but newer fibrates, such as fenofibrate and particularly ciprofibrate, have increased rapidly. Gemfibrozil is now declining in usage. There has been a 70% increase in usage over the past five years, although it has now levelled off. Fibrates now account for 18% of prescriptions for lipid-lowering drugs, but only 10% of the costs.[5] Fibrates have a lower popularity profile than statins and would seem to only infrequently figure in the major clinical trials now.

Antihypertensives

Hypertension is a major risk factor which is amenable to treatment. Thiazide diuretics and β-blockers are the only two groups of drugs for which long-term beneficial effects on morbidity and mortality have been demonstrated. Newer treatments, such as angiotensin converting enzyme (ACE) inhibitors, certainly reduce blood pressure but their long-term effects on morbidity and mortality are not yet known. In the absence of any contraindication to thiazide diuretics or β-blockers, one of these drugs is a rational first choice. Effective treatment at all ages produces a 30% reduction in the risk of coronary artery disease and stroke.[18]

Diuretics

The total usage of diuretics remains constant. The trend is to increased use of thiazides and loop diuretics and a marked reduction in the use of potassium sparing combination diuretics and of diuretics combined with potassium. Research indicates that the optimum antihypertensive effect of thiazide diuretics can be achieved with a maximum of 2.5 mg bendrofluazide.[7] Its use has tripled in the past five years.[5]

ACE inhibitors

ACE inhibitors, in combination with diuretics, can improve the symptoms and prolong the life of many patients with heart failure. They can also be used in the treatment of hypertension. The British Hypertension Society guidelines recommend that the use of ACE inhibitors as first-line therapy should be reserved for those patients whose medical history makes the use of conventional therapies inappropriate.[19] ACE inhibitors should be considered for hypertension when thiazides and β-blockers are contraindicated, not tolerated, or fail to control blood pressure. They are particularly indicated for the treatment of hypertension in insulin-dependant diabetics, but best avoided in patients with renovascular disease, or those who may become pregnant.[7]

The national usage of ACE inhibitors has risen by 250% in the past five years. Captopril, the first ACE inhibitor prescribed for hypertension, is still significantly used, but the main growth in usage has been in enalapril and lisinopril. There is smaller but increasing usage in such drugs as ramipril, fosinopril, and perindopril. Nationally the cost of ACE inhibitors has doubled to £192m/annum in the past five years. The rising cost of the main ACE inhibitors is proportional to their rise in use, as the costs of the three most used drugs are broadly comparable. Currently there is a 2.4-fold variation in the use of these drugs by health authority.[5]

Aims of medical treatment

Medical treatment should aim at greatly improving the patient's quality of life and exercise tolerance. Angina must be kept stable and patients should already be on maximum therapy. Individuals should be referred to a cardiothoracic centre for coronary angiography with a view to coronary angioplasty or bypass surgery.

Conclusion

Patients should understand that medical treatment is not an inferior option in a world of high technology. For single- and two-vessel disease, prognosis on medical treatment is excellent and quality of life is the determining factor in choosing to change to angioplasty or surgery. For patients with three-vessel disease, surgery is more likely to carry a long-term prognostic benefit (as well as symptom relief), especially if left ventricular function is poor. Even clearer is the prognostic advantage of coronary artery bypass grafting over medical treatment in those with significant left main stem vessel disease.

References

1. The NHS Centre for Reviews and Dissemination. *Effective Healthcare bulletin.* York, 1998.
2. Randomized trial of cholesterol lowering in 4,444 patients with coronary heart disease: the Scandinavian Simvastatin Survival Study (4S). *Lancet* 1994; **344**: 1383–9.
3. Shepherd J, Cobbe SM, Ford I *et al.* Prevention of coronary heart disease with pravastatin in men with hyper-cholesterlaemia. *N Engl J Med* 1995; **333**: 1301–7.
4. The Health of the Nation briefing pack 1997. Department of Health.
5. Prescribing analysis and cost (PACT) data 1998. Prescription Pricing Authority.

6. Wassertheil-Smoller S, Oberman A, Blaufox MD *et al*. The trial of antihypertensive interventions and management (TAIM) study. Final results with regard to blood pressure, cardiovascular risk, and quality of life. *Am J Hypertens* 1992; **5**: 37–44.

7. British National Formulary 1998 No 36. British Medical Association and Royal Pharmaceutical Society of Great Britain.

8. Standing medical advisory committee. *The use of statins*. London: 1997.

9. NHS Executive letter (EL (97)41). Statement on use of statins. Department of Health, 1997.

10. Correspondence, Use of statins; *BMJ* 1997; **315**: 1615–20.

11. Ramsey LE, Haq IU, Jackson PR, Yeo WW. The Sheffield table for primary prevention of coronary heart disease. *Lancet* 1996; **348**: 1251–2.

12. Published in a report on the management of mildly raised blood pressure. New Zealand Ministry of Health.

13. The Health of the Nation briefing pack 1991. HMSO.

14. Guidelines for ATC classification and DDD assignment 1996.

15. Sample of prescriptions, 1998. Prescription Pricing Authority.

16. Lloyd DC, Harris CM, Roberts DJ. Specific therapeutic group age-sex related prescribing units (STAR-PUs): weightings for analysing general practices' prescribing in England. *BMJ* 1995; **311**: 991–4.

17. Department of health public health common data set 1995. Institute of public health, University of Surrey.

18. Medical Research Council Working Party. MRC trial of treatment in mild hypertension. *BMJ* 1985; **291**: 97–104.

19. Sever P, Beevers G, Bulpitt C *et al*. Management guidelines in essential hypertension: report of the second working party of the British Hypertension Society. *BMJ* 1993; **306**: 983–7.

Interventional cardiology in unstable angina

Nicholas Curzen, Manchester Heart Centre, Manchester Royal Infirmary
Martin Rothman, London Chest Hospital, London

Unstable angina is one of the most common reasons for hospital admission in the UK.[1–3] This condition and non-Q wave myocardial infarction (MI) are conventionally considered as one heterogeneous patient group. Prognosis for this clinical entity is not benign — within two weeks of diagnosis, acute MI develops in around 12% of patients.[4] Furthermore, patients treated with optimal medical therapy have shown progression rates to fatal or non-fatal MI of 4% and 8% within one year, respectively.[5] Symptoms of unstable angina can be stabilized in approximately 90% of patients by applying aggressive medical therapy including heparin, aspirin, nitrates, β-blockers and calcium channel blockers.[6] New agents that may improve symptom stabilization are currently being assessed.

Who is at greatest risk of further cardiac events?

Clearly, the identification of those patients at greatest risk of further cardiac events, such as fatal or non-fatal MI, represents an important clinical challenge. Such risk stratification has two components. First, and intuitively, the 10% or so of patients whose symptoms and electrocardiogram (ECG) changes do not settle with medical therapy require further assessment and revascularization, both to treat their refractory symptoms and to reduce their risk of future events (which is elevated). The second component is biochemical. Recently, it has become apparent that the underlying pathophysiological mechanism yielding the clinical syndrome of unstable angina involves a localized inflammatory reaction centred on an eroded or fissured plaque featuring platelet aggregation and thrombus formation, and hence restriction of blood flow.[7] Such a dynamic process yields elevated serum concentrations of C-reactive protein (CRP) and, in a proportion of cases, elevation in the level of the cardiac-specific proteins, troponin T and I. The admission level of CRP in patients with unstable angina has been shown to correlate with outcome by more than one group,[8,9] and the level of either troponin T and I also carries prognostic value.[10–3] Since a large proportion of the unstable angina population are likely to come to angiographic assessment and, where appropriate, subsequent revascularization, regardless of the physician's ability to settle the symptoms in the acute phase, the question could be raised: why not perform early angiography on all patients with unstable angina? Such a strategy is inappropriate for two main reasons. Pragmatically, provision of invasive facilities is inadequate to provide such a service. Second, clinical data are available to suggest that the outcome of the population as a whole would be poorer than that achieved using a predominantly conservative strategy. In the Thrombolysis in MI Trial (TIMI IIIB), 1,473 patients with unstable angina or non-Q wave MI were randomized to conservative or invasive strategies following thrombolysis, regardless of symptoms.[14] The combined endpoint consisted of death, further MI or progression to heart failure, and was seen in 18.1% of the conservative group and 16.2% of the invasive group, a difference that was not significant. Similarly, in VANQWISH (Veterans Affairs Non-Q Wave Infarction Strategies in Hospital) study, 920 patients with non-Q wave MI were randomized to conservative or invasive strategies.[15] The in-hospital mortality was higher in the invasive group in this study, although preliminary results from long-term follow-up indicate little difference between the groups. These two studies illustrate the profound difficulty of designing randomized studies in this field: for example, cross-over rates from the conservative to the invasive arms being very high (64% in TIMI IIIB) and the weakness of counting patients who underwent angiography but who were then treated medically as being 'invasive' or 'interventional'. Nevertheless, they sound a loud

39

and clear warning to the aggressive cardiologist or physician that uniform invasive investigation and treatment without regard to symptoms or ischaemic burden is inappropriate and probably harmful. The current recommendation, therefore, is that only the patients at highest risk of further cardiac events should be referred in the early phase for invasive assessment with a view to revascularization.[6] These patients are those with refractory symptoms and/or ischaemia and those with elevated admission levels of troponins or CRP, although the stage of admission of these blood samples may be important.[16]

Percutaneous intervention

Evidence of success

There is some evidence to suggest that the success rate of percutaneous transluminal angioplasty (PTCA), which from now on will be referred to with the implication that stent deployment may also be involved, is lower in patients with unstable angina.[17] These data may, in fact, be out of date given the improvement in equipment and technique that has been seen in the past few years. At the London Chest Hospital, for example, a review of interventional outcome over the period 1 January 1998 to 30 September 1998 demonstrated a success rate of 90.5% (n=147) for unstable cases and 87.1% for stable cases, including chronic total occlusions (n=217). There is no question, however, that the complication rate is higher in the unstable group.[18–20] This is unsurprising in the light of factors such as presence of intracoronary thrombus, rhythm disturbances and haemostatic problems. Nevertheless, it reinforces the need to act only in cases that stand to benefit most from revascularization. Reduction in complication rates from the procedure has been a goal driving much important clinical research, and the increasing use of stents and the selective administration of abciximab are two important (but expensive) tools. The evidence to support the use of stents and abciximab (Reopro) will be discussed in more detail below. First, however, it is important to address the even more taxing question about the evidence to support the use of PTCA in unstable angina at all. There is a paucity of such data. The utilization of percutaneous revascularization techniques has been, and continues to be, symptom- and/or ischaemia-determined. In other words, physicians generally treat their unstable angina patients with maximum medical therapy and refer them for invasive assessment and revascularization only when this strategy fails. Under such circumstances, the forces determining management are dominated by the desire to render the patient asymptomatic so that they may return home. Successful PTCA achieves this objective with considerable efficiency, since most patients will be able to go home within one to two days of the procedure. The success rate of PTCA is, as has already been quoted, over 90%. Thus PTCA offers an efficient, rapid means of symptom relief for most suitable patients, enabling them to return to normal, and freeing up facilities for other patients. The application of such a potent revascularization tool is, therefore, likely to continue to remain widespread, regardless of any prognostic benefit, and will only be reassessed when either concerns regarding possible harmful longer-term effects surface, or another technique renders PTCA obsolete. It would certainly be extremely difficult to set up a randomized trial to test the efficacy of PTCA in patients with refractory unstable angina, since the only two current management alternatives for these highly symptomatic patients would be either medical therapy, which by definition has already failed, and CABG surgery, whose mortality in these circumstances is significantly increased. Thus, the only (indirect) evidence that can be quoted for the benefit of PTCA in unstable angina are outcome data from studies such as EPIC or CAPTURE (discussed below).

Complications

There are two main categories of complications associated with PTCA: short- and longer-term. Short-term complications are dominated by acute vessel closure, either during, immediately after or within 24 hours of the procedure. This has always been a potentially lethal complication of PTCA, but its occurrence is more likely in patients with acute coronary syndromes, whose presentation, as well as other features, such as lesion complexity are known to be factors associated with high risk.[21,22] Acute vessel closure is associated with myocardial infarction, requirement for emergency CABG surgery and death.[17] One of the morphological precursors for vessel occlusion is dissection, and this component can be treated by the deployment of a coronary stent. Stent deployment itself, however, is also associated with vessel thrombosis, a complication which in both stable and unstable patients is reduced by antiplatelet regimens that include ticlopidine and aspirin,[23] but which appears to be specifically reduced in the unstable setting by the administration of abciximab (discussed below). Longer-term complications of PTCA are dominated by restenosis. In unstable patients, restenosis rates can be attenuated by implantation of coronary stents, as in stable patients. For example, in the BENESTENT[24] and STRESS[25] studies, restenosis rates with and without stents were 22% vs 32% and 32% vs 42%, respectively. It appears that stents achieve this lower rate of restenosis by improving the acute gain in vessel diameter at the site of the coronary lesion. Increasing knowledge regarding this process has helped to focus stent deployment still further, so that more recent data now suggest that careful deployment of stents can yield restenosis rates as low as 10–15%.[26]

Abciximab (Reopro)

The intensive search for therapeutic weapons with which to fight complications of PTCA has so far produced the antiplatelet agent, abciximab (Reopro, Eli Lilly). As has already been discussed, a primary element in the pathophysiology of acute coronary syndromes is platelet aggregation. In addition, acute vessel occlusion and stent thrombosis represent an important reason for complications in PTCA. The final common pathway for platelet aggregation is the binding of the glycoprotein receptor complex, GP IIb/IIIa, to fibrinogen.[27,28] Increased expression of GP IIb/IIIa receptors is, therefore, a fundamental step in the process leading to platelet aggregation. and this can be stimulated by a variety of mechanisms, only some of which are inhibited by agents such as aspirin. Abciximab is the Fab fragment of a human-murine chimeric antibody (c7E3) which occupies the GP IIb/IIIa platelet receptors, thereby blocking the mechanism for aggregation. Several studies have now been carried out that, particularly when analysed as a group, provide powerful evidence for the administration of abciximab in high risk PTCA procedures. As a result of these data, abciximab is increasingly used in procedures involving patients with unstable coronary syndromes in order to reduce complication rates. These trials are summarized below.

In the EPIC study, 2,099 patients undergoing high risk PTCA/ atherectomy were recruited.[29] Patients were randomized to receive Reopro bolus (0.25mg/kg) + infusion 10μg/min for 12 hours) or placebo bolus and infusion in addition to routine aspirin and heparin therapy. The composite endpoint consisted of death, non-fatal MI and requirement for urgent revascularization. The results demonstrated a significant reduction in the composite endpoint at 30 days, six months and three years (Table 1). The investigators were therefore able to conclude that there was a significant and long-lasting reduction in complications with abciximab in these high-risk patients. It is, perhaps, worth noting that only seven patients in the whole study received a stent, hence making the applicability of these data to current practice (in which stent rates are up to 90% in some centres) less clear cut.

In EPILOG,[30] 2,792 patients were included who were undergoing urgent or elective PTCA. Patients were randomized to receive: Reopro bolus (0.25mg/kg) followed by an infusion (0.125μg/kg/min for 12 hours) in combination with standard dose heparin (100U/kg or maximum 10,000U); or Reopro bolus (0.25mg/kg) followed by an infusion (0.125μg/kg/min

Table 1 Number of deaths, non-MI cases and need for revascularization following the EPIC Study[28]

Endpoint	30 days	6 months	3 years
Placebo	12.8%	35.1%	47.2%
Reopro	8.3%	27%	41.1%
p value	0.008	0.001	0.009

for 12 hours) in combination with weight-adjusted heparin (70U/kg, maximum 7,000U); or placebo bolus and infusion with standard dose heparin (100U/kg or maximum 10,000U). Again, the composite endpoint was made up of death, MI and need for urgent intervention. The results yielded two main conclusions (Table 2). First, that abciximab reduced the risk of acute ischaemic complications of PTCA in this population. Second, the occurrence of significant haemorrhagic complications in this context could be limited to the same degree as that seen with routine heparin therapy without abciximab, if abciximab was employed with weight-adjusted heparin (70U/kg).

The third important abciximab study was called CAPTURE.[31] In this study, there were 1,265 patients with refractory unstable angina. In order to be included into the study, these patients underwent angiography. Those in whom PTCA was deemed suitable therapy were then randomized to receive either: planned treated with abciximab bolus (0.25mg/kg) followed by an infusion (10μg/min) for 18–24hrs prior to intervention + 1 hr afterwards; or placebo bolus and infusion. The composite endpoint was represented by the combination of death, MI and need for urgent intervention. This study again found a significant reduction in the endpoint at three months, 15.9% in the placebo group versus 11.3% in the abciximab group ($p=0.012$). Interestingly, however, this beneficial endpoint reduction was not preserved at the six-month follow-up time point, when both groups had a 30.8% endpoint. This result has lead to speculation that the abciximab infusion after the procedure (as in EPIC and EPILOG) is an important component of its beneficial effect in the longer term.

Stent use

As has already been implied, one of the major difficulties in extrapolating the results of EPIC and EPILOG, in particular, to current practice is that these two studies included only seven and 382 patients in whom stents were implanted, respectively. The current stenting rate at the London Chest Hospital is just over 90%. Further data are therefore required to help establish whether or not the benefits of abciximab in patients undergoing balloon angioplasty only (POBA) are also available to a population of patients undergoing stent deployment. Recent publication of the EPISTENT Study[32] has gone some way to answer this question, although not specifically in the context of unstable angina. EPISTENT recruited 2,399 patients with ischaemic heart disease and coronary anatomy suitable for PTCA. These patients were then randomized to three groups: Stent plus placebo; stent plus abciximab; and POBA plus abciximab. Abciximab was administered as a bolus (0.25mg/kg) up to one hour before intervention, followed by an infusion of 0.125μg/kg/min for 12 hours. Again the composite endpoint was represented by death, MI and need for urgent revascularization. The 30-day outcome results are summarized in Table 3. They demonstrate a significant reduction in endpoint frequency in both the abciximab groups when compared to the stent plus placebo group, the stent plus abciximab group having the lowest rate of all. The two conclusions from these data were as follows: first that abciximab substantially improves the safety of coronary stenting procedures, and second that balloon angioplasty with abciximab is safer than stenting without abciximab. The contentious speculation arising from this study has, of course, been that there is an argument for treating all patients who undergo PTCA with abciximab! Clearly further data are required, specifically with longer-term follow-up.

Regardless of the debate concerning the more general indications for GPIIb/IIIa antibodies/inhibitors, current clinical practice reflects the data suggesting a significant reduction in complications in patients undergoing PTCA who are at high risk. By currently defined risk

Table 2 Number of deaths, non-MI cases and need for revascularization in the EPILOG Study[29]

Endpoint	30 days	6 months
Placebo	11.7%	25.8%
Reopro+ standard heparin	5.4%	22.3%
p value (vs placebo)	<0.001	0.04
Reopro + wt-adjusted heparin	5.2%	22.8%
p value (vs placebo)	<0.001	0.07

Table 3 Results of the EPISTENT Study[32]

	30-day outcome	*p* value (vs placebo)
Stent + placebo	10.8%	
Stent + reopro	5.3%	<0.001
POBA + reopro	6.9%	0.007

stratification data,[17,21,22] many patients with unstable angina, especially those with complex coronary lesion morphology or thrombus have a clear-cut indication for abciximab and its administration is virtually routine for this sub-population. It may be that in the future, it will be possible to identify patients, who by virtue of their genotype, are at higher than normal risk of complications such as stent thrombosis.[33–35] Such precision in risk stratification leads to the prospect of tailoring therapy such as GPIIb/IIIa blockade to those who specifically require it.

Conclusion

Unstable angina and non-Q wave MI are two of the most common reasons for medical admission, providing a significant risk of progression to MI or death. Unstable angina patients at greatest risk of progressing to MI or death are those unable to settle on optimal medical therapy and those with elevated levels of C-reactive protein and troponins T and I. These patients should, therefore, be referred for early angiographic assessment with a view to revascularization.

One such technique is PTCA. This procedure (with or without stenting) is highly effective in such treatment, but is associated with several complications, such as acute vessel closure, stent thrombosis and, in the longer term, restenosis. Although stategies are available for reducing such complications, further research is required to determine whether or not PTCA definitely improves prognosis in these circumstances.

References

1. *Acute Care Statistics 1996*. CHKS Ltd, Alcester, Warwickshire: Health Resource Groups National Statistics 1995/6.
2. Purcell H. The epidemiology of unstable angina. *Br J Cardiol* 1998; **5**(suppl 2): S3–4.
3. Bowker T, Turner B, Roberts T *et al*, for the SAMII group. Is the occurrence, management and outcome of acute myocardial ischaemia and infarction gender dependent? *J Am Coll Cardiol* 1998; **31**(2, suppl A): 524A.
4. American Heart Association. *Heart and Stroke Facts*. Dallas, Texas: American Heart Association National Center, 1996.
5. Davies MJ. The role of plaque pathology in coronary thrombosis. *Clin Cardiol* 1997; **20**(suppl 1): 1–7.
6. Campbell RWF, Wallentin L, Verheught FWA *et al*. Management strategies for a better outcome in unstable coronary artery disease. *Clin Cardiol* 1998; **21**: 314–22.
7. Neuhaus KL. Cornary thrombosis — defining the goals, improving the outcome. *Clin Cardiol* 1997; **20**(suppl 1): 8–13.
8. Liuzzo G, Biasucci LM, Gallimore JR *et al*. The prognostic value of C-reactive protein and serum amyloid A protein in severe unstable angina. *N Engl J Med* 1994; **331**: 417–24.
9. Haverkate F, Thompson SG, Pyke SDM *et al*. Production of C-reactive protein and risk of coronary events in stable and unstable angina. *Lancet* 1997; **349**: 462–6.
10. Hamm CW, Ravkilde J, Gerhardt W *et al*. The prognostic value of serum troponin T in unstable angina. *N Engl J Med* 1992; **327**: 146–50.
11. Ohman EM, Armstrong PW, Christensen RH *et al*. Cardiac troponin T levels for risk stratification in acute myocardial ischemia. *N Engl J Med* 1996; **335**: 1333–41.
12. Antman EM, Tansijevic MJ, Thompson B *et al*. Cardiac-specific troponin I levels to predict the risk of mortality in patients with acute coronary syndromes. *N Engl J Med* 1996; **335**: 1342–9.
13. Lindhal B, Venge P, Wallentin L. Relation between troponin T and subsequent cardiac events in unstable coronary artery disease. *Circulation* 1996; **93**: 1651–7.
14. Langer A, Goodman SG, Topol E *et al*. Late assessment of thrombolytic efficacy (LATE) study: prognosis in patients with non-Q wave myocardial infarction. *J Am Coll Cardiol* 1996; **27**: 1327–32.

15. The bypass angioplasty revascularization investigation (BARI) Investigators: comparison of coronary bypass surgery with angioplasty in patients with multivessel disease. *N Engl J Med* 1996; **335**: 217–25.

16. De Feyter PJ. The benefits and risks of coronary intervention — balancing the equation. *Clin Cardiol* 1997; **20**(suppl 1): 14–21.

17. Stammen F, De Scheerder I, Glazier JJ et al. Immediate and follow-up results of the conservative coronary angioplasty strategy for unstable angina pectoris. *Am J Cardiol* 1992; **69**: 1533–7.

18. De Feyter PJ, Serruys PW, van den Brand M, Hugenholtz PG. Percutaneous transluminal coronary angioplasty for unstable angina. *Am J Cardiol* 1991; **68**(suppl B): 125B-35B.

19. Detre K, Holubkov R, Kelsey S et al. The National Heart, Lung & Blood Institute's Percutaneous Transluminal Coronary Angioplasty Registry: PTCA in 1985–1986 and 1977–1981. *N Engl J Med* 1988; **318**: 265–70.

20. Ellis SG, Bates ER, Schaible T et al. Prospects for the use of antagonists to the platelet glycoprotein IIb/IIIa receptor to prevent post-angioplasty restenosis and thrombosis. *J Am Coll Cardiol* 1991; **17**(suppl B): 89B-95B.

21. De Feyter PJ, Ruygrok PN. Coronary intervention: risk stratification and management of abrupt coronary occlusion. *Eur Heart J* 1995; **16**(suppl L): L97-L103.

22. Schomig A, Neumann FJ, Kastrati A et al. A randomized comparison of antiplatelet and anticoagulation therapy after the placement of coronary artery stents. *N Engl J Med* 1996; **334**: 1084–9.

23. Serruys PW, de Jaegere P, Kiemeneij F et al. A comparison of balloonÔexpandable stent implantation with balloon angioplasty in patients with coronary artery disease. *N Engl J Med* 1994; **331**: 489–95.

24. Fischman DL, Leon MB, Baim DS et al. A randomized comparison of coronary stent placement and balloon angioplasty in the treatment of coronary disease. *N Engl J Med* 1994; **331**: 496–501.

25. De Jaegere P, Mudra H, Almagor Y et al. Intravascular ultrasound-guided optimized stent deployment. Immediate and six months clinical and angiographic results from the Multicentre Ultrasound Stenting in Coronaries Study (MUSIC). *Eur Heart J* 1998; **19**: 1214–23.

26. Leftowitz RJ, Plow EF, Topol EJ. Platelet glycoprotein IIb/IIIa receptors in cardiovascular medicine. *N Engl J Med* 1995; **332**: 1553–9.

27. Idker PM, Hennekens CH, Schmitz et al. PIA1/A2 polymorphism of platelet glycoprotein IIIa and risks of myocardial infarction, stroke and venous thrombosis. *Lancet* 1997; **349**: 385–8.

28. The EPIC Investigators. Use of a monoclonal antibody directed against the platelet glycoprotein IIb/IIIa receptor in high risk coronary angioplasty. *N Engl J Med* 1994; **330**: 956–61.

29. Topol EJ, califf RM, Lincoff AM et al, for the EPILOG investigators. Platelet glycoprotein IIb/IIIa receptor blockade and low dose heparin during percutaneous coronary revascularization. *N Engl J Med* 1997; **336**: 1689–96.

30. The CAPTURE Investigators. Randomized placebo-controlled trial of abciximab before and during coronary intervention in refractory unstable angina: The CAPTURE study. *Lancet* 1997; **349**: 1429–35.

31. The EPISTENT Investigators. Randomized placebo-controlled and balloon-angioplasty-controlled trial to assess safety of coronary stenting with use of glycoprotein IIb/IIIa blockade. *Lancet* 1998; **352**: 87–92.

32. Curzen NP, Goodall AH, Hurd C et al. Stimulated platelets of patients with the PIA2 allele for platelet membrane GP111a exhibit increased fibrinogen binding. *Eur Heart J* 1998; **19**(suppl): 360.

33. Goodhall A, Curzen N, Hurd C et al. Increased binding of fibrinogen to glycoprotein IIIa-proline 33 (HPA-1b), PIA2, Zwb) positive platelets in patients with cardiovascular disease. *Eur Heart J* 1999; **20**(10): 742–7.

34. Wiss EJ, Bray PF, Tayback M et al. A polymorphism of a platelet glycoprotein receptor is an inherited risk factor for coronary thrombosis. *N Engl J Med* 1996; **334**: 1090–4.

35. Walter DH, Schachinger V, Elsner M et al. Platelet glycoprotein IIIa polymorphisms and risk of coronary stent thrombosis. *Lancet* 1997; **350**: 1217–9.

Role of surgery in the management of unstable coronary artery disease

John Dunning, Cardiothoracic Surgery Department, Papworth Hospital NHS Trust, Cambridge

Unstable coronary artery disease (CAD) is a term encompassing both unstable angina and non-Q wave myocardial infarction (MI). The main event in initiating this acute clinical syndrome is fissuring or rupture of an atheromatous plaque and the formation of a platelet-rich mural thrombus.[1] This results in either partial or transient occlusion of the coronary artery, compounded by embolization of platelets into the distal myocardial vessels and coronary artery spasm.

Management of CAD continues to present a major challenge to clinicians. Even with appropriate treatment, the risk of MI or death may be as high as 10% within the first six weeks of presentation.[2,3] Major advances have been made in acute medical, interventional and surgical therapy, however, the optimal management strategy for these patients is still being debated, influenced by comparative results and cost implications. This paper will discuss the indications and timing of surgery, and consider the outcome following operation in patients with unstable CAD. Controversies regarding the concept of early revascularization versus medical therapy, and comparative outcomes of percutaneous transluminal coronary angioplasty (PTCA) and surgery will also be addressed.

Current medical therapy

Major advances in the acute medical therapy of patients with unstable CAD have taken place over the past 20 years. Initial therapy is based on the reversal of thrombus formation and artery occlusion. Anti-ischaemic therapy includes intravenous nitrates and selective β-blockade. Calcium channel blockers, such as diltiazem and verapamil, reduce the frequency of anginal attacks; verapamil, however, is contraindicated in patients with impaired left ventricular function or with concomitant β-blockade. Neither drug should be used in patients suffering from disorders of cardiac conduction.[4]

Aspirin inhibits the action of the prostaglandin thromboxane A_2 — this, in turn, inhibits platelet activation and thrombus formation, thereby improving survival in patients with unstable CAD.[5]

Glycoprotein IIb/IIIa receptor antagonists, such as abciximab (Reopro), also inhibit platelet aggregation and the EPIC and CAPTURE studies have shown that these drugs reduce MI and the incidence of death.[6,7] Abciximab is often given with aspirin and heparin. Other antiplatelet drugs, such as clopidogrel, are currently under investigation but not yet licensed for use in the UK.

Unfractionated heparins have played a central role in the acute management of unstable CAD. However, low molecular weight heparins, such as enoxaparin, have a more predictable anticoagulant effect and have been shown to reduce the incidence of death, MI and recurrent angina (as a combined endpoint) compared to conventional, unfractionated heparin infusion.[8]

Thrombolytic therapy is associated with a poorer outcome than placebo in unstable CAD patients and is contraindicated in this syndrome.[3]

Surgical revascularization

Indications for surgery

The indications for surgical revascularization in patients with unstable CAD have been derived from the results of randomized studies and, more recently, a number of non-randomized protocols.

Two major, multicentre, randomized trials comparing surgical versus medical therapy for unstable angina were undertaken in the 1970s. First, the National Heart, Lung and Blood Institute-sponsored National Cooperative Study Group trial included 288 patients with unstable angina who had initially been treated with medical therapy between 1972 and 1976.[9,10] This study showed two-year survival to be similar between the groups (90% and 91% for medical and surgical therapy respectively), while the incidence of non-fatal MI was higher in the surgical group (17% versus 8%). The incidence of severe angina pectoris, however, was significantly reduced in the surgical group at one year and 31% of patients originally assigned to medical therapy underwent surgery by two years. Second, the Veterans Administration study included 468 male patients with unstable angina between 1976 and 1982.[11–4] Five-year mortality demonstrated a clear survival advantage in patients with triple-vessel disease undergoing surgery (89% versus 76%). Patients with impaired left ventricular ejection fraction also gained particular benefit from surgery.[11–4]

Although these studies are important, they are very limited as a result of their comparison of outdated medical and surgical protocols. In particular, the advantages of antiplatelet and anti-thrombotic therapy, advances in myocardial protection regimen and the influence of internal mammary artery use have not been measured. In addition, the studies exclude patients with left main stem stenosis, previous coronary artery surgery and postinfarction angina.

A number of non-randomized studies have more recently been carried out to determine the outcome of surgery in patients with post-MI unstable angina. For example, Lee *et al* studied 1,181 consecutive patients who had undergone isolated coronary revascularization between 1992 and 1995.[15] This group consisted of 865 patients who had never had MI and 316 who had recently (< 21 days ago) suffered MI — the latter group were subdivided into four groups according to increasing clinical severity (Table 1). Mortality in the non-MI group was 2.5% while in patients with previous MI, mortality increased from 1.2% in stable angina patients to 26% in patients experiencing cardiogenic shock. Multivariate logistic regression analysis identified left ventricular dysfunction, intra-aortic balloon pump pulsation and renal insufficiency as the only independent predictors of mortality. Other studies have confirmed the higher risk of surgery in patients with post-MI unstable angina and impaired left ventricular function.[16,17]

Appropriate timing

The timing of surgery following MI has also been studied. Curtis *et al* studied 993 consecutive patients undergoing coronary artery bypass grafting for postinfarction unstable angina.[18] Patients were divided into five groups according to the time period between MI and surgery. Operative mortality was lowest when surgery was performed three weeks to three months after MI, and highest when surgery was carried out soon after presentation (Table 2).

Table 1 Mortality risk for post-infarct unstable angina patients following coronary artery bypass surgery[15]

Clinical Severity	Number	% mortality
Non-MI	865	2.5
Post MI:		
Stable angina	166	1.2
Unstable angina	107	3.7
Intra-aortic balloon pump support	20	8.0
Cardiogenic shock	23	26.0

Early angiography and revascularization versus conservative therapy

Although acute medical treatment controls symptoms and reverses ischaemic changes in most unstable CAD patients, the appropriate management of these stabilized patients remains controversial.

The conservative approach to management involves mobilization, hospital discharge and outpatient follow-up. Concerns about one such approach, however, have arisen from observations that patients with unstable CAD have a much higher risk of suffering adverse events, such as MI or unstable angina (57% versus 17% for stable patients).[19] In one study, for example, 31% of 85 patients with stabilized angina suffered a serious adverse event — one death and 25 non-fatal coronary events. Nearly 56% of the clinical events were related to progression of ischaemia-related stenoses.

A more aggressive means of management involving early angiography and revascularization is favoured by some. Two large randomized trials compared the strategy of early intervention (PTCA or surgery) with conservative therapy.[3,20] The Veterans Affairs Non-Q Wave Infarction Strategies in Hospital (VANQWISH) trial, which included 920 patients, revealed the number of patients suffering the combined endpoint of death or non-fatal MI, or death alone to be significantly higher in the early intervention group at one-month post-intervention and at one-year follow-up. Of those patients undergoing coronary artery bypass surgery, the 30-day mortality was 11.6% in the early intervention group and 3.4% in the group treated conservatively in the first instance. This study suggests that a conservative approach may be safer than an early intervention strategy.

The Thrombolysis in MI trial (TIMI IIIB) randomized 1,473 patients. When strategies for early invasive versus conservative treatment were studied, the combined incidence of death, MI or recurrent pain at six weeks were found to be similar (16.2% versus 18.1% respectively).

Thus, early intervention does not seem to be appropriate in patients whose symptoms are stabilized by acute medical therapy. For patients whose symptoms do not settle within 48 hours, however, urgent angiography and revascularization is warranted. Risk stratification may be an effective clinical means of identifying patients at great risk of adverse events despite resolution of signs of ischaemia with medical therapy. Factors predictive of adverse outcome following an unstable episode include elderly patients (ie > 70 years), persisting ST changes, elevated biochemical markers (creatinine kinase isoforms and troponins) and recent MI.[21]

Surgical revascularization versus percutaneous transluminal coronary angioplasty

Several randomized trials comparing coronary artery bypass grafting and PTCA have been undertaken — at least four have included a large proportion of patients with unstable angina.[22-5] No trial has, to date, demonstrated any mortality difference between surgery and PTCA in the overall group of patients studied. However, the Bypass and Angioplasty Revascularization Investigation (BARI) trial demonstrated reduced mortality in diabetic patients undergoing hypoglycaemic therapy at five years. This has major implications for surgical practice in the future which will comprise more diabetic patients with small, severely diseased, coronary arteries.

The most striking differences found between the two procedures are the completeness of revascularization and incidence of restenosis. In the Emory Angioplasty versus Surgery Trial (EAST)[24] and ERACI (an Argentine trial)[25] trials, complete revascularization was achieved only in 75% and 51% of the PTCA

Table 2 Mortality risk for coronary artery bypass surgery in relation to time following MI[18]

Time period between MI and surgery	% mortality
0–24 hours	18.6
1–7 days	7.4
1–3 weeks	5.9
3 weeks to 3 months	2.7

patients respectively, compared with 99% and 88% respectively in the surgical group. The greatest limitation of PTCA is its high restenosis rate, which accounts for the increased number of repeat procedures in Table 3.

Can we improve outcome?

Although surgery performed on patients with unstable CAD produces excellent long-term results, early mortality is higher than that following surgery for stable angina. A study by Louagie et al involved 474 patients with unstable angina who underwent coronary artery bypass surgery from 1986 to 1993.[26] Revascularization in these patients included the use of saphenous veins and multiple arterial conduits. The duration of aortic cross clamping was found to be the main predictor of death and low-cardiac output. These observations suggest that preservation of the ischaemic myocardium is paramount to a successful outcome for surgery in patients with unstable CAD. Other adverse factors included: female sex, the presence of left ventricular aneurysm, the number of diseased vessels and re-operation. In addition, haemodynamic data demonstrated a significantly reduced left ventricular stroke work index and higher pulmonary vascular resistance in patients with poor outcome following surgery.

Cold blood cardioplegia has been shown to reduce morbidity and mortality in patients undergoing urgent coronary artery bypass grafting for unstable angina.[27,28] Further advances in cardioplegic protocol, such as warm blood cardioplegic induction and multidose cold cardioplegia for maintenance and controlled reperfusion, have been shown to improve mortality in patients with acute coronary occlusion.[29]

Internal mammary artery conduit use in surgery has now been widely experienced, but its suitability in emergency situations is not uniformly accepted. Technical considerations are not legitimate reasons for avoiding its use in emergency cases, but the increased risks of postoperative spasm in such conduits may be more relevant.Studies have shown that internal mammary artery use is not associated with increased complications[30] and, infact, increased operative mortality[17] and low-cardiac output state[31] have been predicted when this conduit is not used, although these observations may be explained by the selection of lower risk cases.

Surgery in the elderly

Much attention has recently been given to the treatment of unstable angina in the elderly following an increase in the number of older patients presenting to clinicians. Vassilikos et al found improved long-term outcome following coronary artery bypass surgery in 60 patients

Table 3 Randomized trials comparing coronary artery bypass surgery with PTCA

	Trial			
	BARI	**RITA**	**EAST**	**ERACI**
Number of patients	1,829	1,011	392	127
Study period	1988–91	1988–91	1987–90	1988–90
Unstable angina cases (%)	70	59	60	83
One-year mortality (%)				
Surgery	10.7*	1.2	2.1	4.7
PTCA	13.7	1.8	3.5	4.8
Repeat procedures (%)				
Surgery	8	5	22	3
PTCA	54	30	41	32

* Five-year mortality

compared with 49 patients undergoing PTCA,[32] although surgery was found to be associated with higher mortality (10% versus 4% in the PTCA group). Authors of this study suggest that elderly patients fit for surgery should not be denied the benefits of revascularization by this means. Eggeling *et al* demonstrated comparable short- and long-term mortality in patients over 75 years with unstable angina treated by surgery or PTCA (6% versus 4% respectively, short term; 4% versus 8% respectively, mean 28 months).[33] As before, the number of repeat procedures and recurrence of angina was higher in the PTCA group. A prospective, multi-centre, randomized trial (AWESOME) of coronary artery bypass surgery and PTCA, which includes patients ≥70 years, is currently being conducted.

Conclusion

Current acute medical therapy resolves ischaemia in most patients presenting with unstable CAD. There is no evidence to support early intervention in those whose symptoms improve with pharmacological treatment, but continued ischaemia (> 48 hours) is an urgent indication for coronary angiography and revascularization.

Coronary artery surgery is more beneficial than medical therapy to triple-vessel coronary heart disease patients and to those with impaired left ventricular ejection fraction. Patients with postinfarction angina and preserved left ventricular function also show positive results following surgery.

Although surgery and PTCA are both associated with higher morbidity and mortality rates when performed on unstable angina patients, surgery has been shown to have a greater survival benefit in diabetic patients than PTCA. The very high incidence of restenosis and incomplete revascularization associated with PTCA limit its efficacy. However, the higher incidence of peri-operative MI observed in patients with unstable CAD who undergo surgery indicates that PTCA continues to have a role in the treatment of these individuals, perhaps as a bridge to surgery. Advances in myocardial preservation techniques, the use of beating heart surgery (without circulatory support by cardiopulmonary bypass) and the wider application of arterial conduits may help to reduce the peri-operative risks in these patients in the future.

References

1. Kristensen S, Ravn H, Falk E. Insights into the pathophysiology of unstable coronary artery disease. *Am J Cardiol* 1997; **80**(5A): 5E-9E.

2. Fragmin during instability in Coronary Artery Disease (FRISC) study group. Low-molecular-weight heparin during instability in coronary artery disease. *Lancet* 1996; **347**: 561–8.

3. The TIMI IIIB Investigators. Effects of tissue plasminogen activator and a comparison of early invasive and conservative strategies in unstable angina and non-Q wave myocardial infarction. Results of the TIMI IIIB trial. *Circulation* 1994; **89**: 1545–56.

4. Anonymous. Management of unstable angina. *Drug Ther Bull* 1998; **36**(5): 36–9.

5. Antiplatelet Trialists' Collaboration. Collaborative overview of randomised trials of antiplatelet therapy-I: prevention of death, myocardial infarction, and stroke by prolonged antiplatelet therapy in various categories of patients. *BMJ* 1994; **308**: 81–106.

6. Lincoff A, Califf R, Anderson K *et al*, for the EPIC Investigators. Evidence for prevention of death and myocardial infarction with platelet membrane glycoprotein IIb/IIIa receptor blockade by abciximab (c7E3 Fab) among patients with unstable angina undergoing percutaneous coronary revascularization. *J Am Coll Cardiol* 1997; **30**: 149–56.

7. The CAPTURE Investigators. Randomised placebo-controlled trial of abciximab before and during coronary intervention in refractory unstable angina: the CAPTURE study. *Lancet* 1997; **349**: 1429–35.

8. Cohen M, Demers C, Gurfinkel E *et al*, for the Efficacy and Safety of Subcutaneous Enoxaparin in Non-Q Wave Coronary Events Study Group. A comparison of low-molecular-weight heparin with unfractionated heparin for unstable coronary artery disease. *N Engl J Med* 1997; **337**: 447–52.

9. Unstable Angina Pectoris Study Group. Unstable angina pectoris national cooperative study group to compare surgical and medical therapy: II. In-hospital experience and initial follow-up results in patients with one, two and three vessel disease. *Am J Cardiol* 1978; **42**: 839–48.

10. Unstable Angina Pectoris Study Group. Unstable angina pectoris national cooperative study group to compare surgical and medical therapy: III. Results in patients with ST segment elevation during pain. *Am J Cardiol* 1980; **45**: 819–24.

11. Luchi R, Scott S, Deupress R and the Principal Investigators and Their Associates of Veterans Administration Cooperative Study No 28. Comparison of medical and surgical treatment for unstable angina pectoris. Results of a Veterans Administration Cooperative study. *N Engl J Med* 1987; **316**: 977–84.

12. Scott S, Luchi R, Deupree R and the Veterans Administration Unstable Angina Cooperative Study Group. Veterans Administration Cooperative Study for treatment of patients with unstable angina. Results in patients with abnormal left ventricular function. *Circulation* 1988; **78**(Suppl I): I113–21.

13. Parisi A, Khuri S, Deupree R *et al*. Medical compared with surgical management of unstable angina five-year mortality and morbidity in the Veterans Administration study. *Circulation* 1989; **80**: 1176–89.

14. Sharma G, Deupree R, Khuri S *et al*. Coronary bypass surgery improves survival in high-risk unstable angina. Results of a Veterans Administration Cooperative study with an eight-year follow-up. *Circulation* 1991; **84**(Suppl III): III260–7.

15. Lee J, Murrell H, Strony J *et al*. Risk analysis of coronary bypass surgery after acute myocardial infarction. *Surgery* 1997; **122**: 675–81.

16. Jones R, Pifarre R, Sullivan H *et al*. Early myocardial revascularization for postinfarction angina. *Ann Thorac Surg* 1987; **44**: 159–63.

17. Fremes S, Goldman B, Weisel R *et al*. Recent preoperative myocardial infarction increases the risk of surgery for unstable angina. *J Cardiovasc Surg* 1991; **6**: 2–12.

18. Curtis J, Walls J, Salam N *et al*. Impact of unstable angina on operative mortality with coronary revascularization at varying time intervals after myocardial infarction. *J Thorac Cardiovasc Surg* 1991; **102**: 867–73.

19. Chester M, Chen L, Kaski J. Angiographic stenosis progression and coronary events in patients with 'stabilised' unstable angina. *Br Heart J* 1995; **91**: 2319–24.

20. Boden W, O'Rourke R, Crawford M for the Veterans Affairs Non-Q Wave Infarction Strategies in Hospital (VANQWISH) Trial Investigators. Outcomes in patients with acute non-Q wave myocardial infarction randomly assigned to an invasive as compared with a conservative management strategy. *N Engl J Med* 1998; **338**: 1785–92.

21. Campbell R, Wallentin L, Verheught F *et al*. Management strategies for a better outcome in unstable coronary artery disease. *Clin Cardiol* 1998; **21**: 314–22.

22. The Bypass and Angioplasty Revascularization Investigation (BARI) Investigators. Comparison of coronary bypass surgery with angioplasty in patients with multivessel disease. *N Engl J Med* 1996; **335**(4): 217–25.

23. RITA Trial Participants. Coronary angioplasty versus coronary artery bypass surgery: the Randomised Intervention Treatment of Angina (RITA) trial. *Lancet* 1993; **341**: 573–80.

24. King S, Lembo N, Weintraub W *et al*. A randomised trial comparing coronary angioplasty with coronary bypass surgery. *N Engl J Med* 1994; **331**: 1044–50.

25. Rodriguez A, Boullon F, Perez-Balino N *et al*. Argentine randomised trial of percutaneous transluminal coronary angioplasty versus coronary artery bypass surgery in multivessel disease (ERACI): in-hospital results and 1-year follow-up. *J Am Coll Cardiol* 1993; **22**: 1060–7.

26. Louagie Y, Jamart J, Buche M *et al*. Operation for unstable angina pectoris: factors influencing adverse in-hospital outcome. *Ann Thorac Surg* 1995; **59**: 1141–9.

27. Christakis G, Fremes S, Weisel R *et al*. Reducing the risk of urgent revascularization for unstable angina: a randomised clinical trial. *J Vasc Surg* 1986; **3**: 764–72.

28. Teoh K, Christakis G, Weisel R *et al*. Increased risk of urgent *revascularization*. *J Thorac Cardiovasc Surg* 1987; **93**: 291–9.

29. Beyersdorf F, Mitrev Z, Sarai K *et al*. Changing patterns of patients undergoing emergency surgical *revascularization* for acute coronary occlusion. Importance of myocardial protection techniques. *J Thorac Cardiovasc Surg* 1993; **106**: 137–48.

30. Edwards F, Bellamy R, Burge J *et al*. True emergency coronary artery bypass surgery. *Ann Thorac Surg* 1990; **49**: 603–11.

31. Elami A, Merin G, Shushan Y. Use of the internal mammary artery for urgent myocardial revascularization. *Cardiovasc Surg* 1993; **1**: 276–9.

32. Vassilikos V, Lim R, Kreidieh I *et al*. Myocardial revascularization in elderly patients with refractory or unstable angina and advanced coronary disease. *Coron Artery Dis* 1997; **8**: 705–09.

33. Eggeling T, Holz W, Osterhues H *et al*. Management of unstable angina in patients over 75 years old. *Coron Artery Dis* 1995; **6**: 891–6.

Index